T0295442

SPINAL FUSION TECHNIQUES

Other books in this series

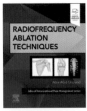 Alaa Abd-Elsayed, Radiofrequency Ablation Techniques, 1e
ISBN: 9780323870634

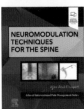 Alaa Abd-Elsayed, Neuromodulation Techniques for the Spine, 1e
ISBN: 9780323875844

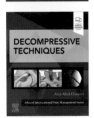 Alaa Abd-Elsayed, Decompressive Techniques, 1e
ISBN : 9780323877510

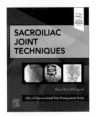 Alaa Abd-Elsayed, Sacroiliac Joint Techniques, 1e
ISBN: 9780323877541

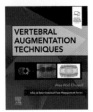 Alaa Abd-Elsayed, Vertebral Augmentation Techniques, 1e
ISBN: 9780323882262

SPINAL FUSION TECHNIQUES

Atlas of Interventional Pain Management Series

Alaa Abd-Elsayed, MD, MPH, CPE, FASA

Medical Director, UW Health Pain Services
Medical Director, UW Pain Clinic
Division Chief, Chronic Pain Management
Department of Anesthesiology
University of Wisconsin
Madison, Wisconsin
United States

ELSEVIER

Elsevier
1600 John F. Kennedy Blvd.
Ste 1800
Philadelphia, PA 19103-2899

Spinal Fusion Techniques   ISBN: 978-0-323-88223-1
Atlas of Interventional Pain Management Series
Copyright © 2024 by Elsevier Inc. All rights reserved.

Notice

Practitioners and researchers must always rely on their own experience and knowledge in evaluating and using any information, methods, compounds or experiments described herein. Because of rapid advances in the medical sciences, in particular, independent verification of diagnoses and drug dosages should be made. To the fullest extent of the law, no responsibility is assumed by Elsevier, authors, editors or contributors for any injury and/or damage to persons or property as a matter of products liability, negligence or otherwise, or from any use or operation of any methods, products, instructions, or ideas contained in the material herein.

Senior Content Development Manager: Somodatta Roy Choudhury
Executive Content Strategist: Michael Houston
Senior Content Development Specialist: Malvika Shah
Publishing Services Manager: Shereen Jameel
Project Manager: Maria Shalini
Senior Designer: Patrick C. Ferguson

Printed in India

Last digit is the print number: 9 8 7 6 5 4 3 2 1

Working together to grow libraries in developing countries

www.elsevier.com • www.bookaid.org

Dedication

To my God, my parents, my wife, and my two beautiful kids Maro and George.

Contributors

Alaa Abd-Elsayed, MD, MPH, CPE, FASA
Medical Director, UW Health Pain Services
Medical Director, UW Pain Clinic
Division Chief, Chronic Pain Management
Department of Anesthesiology
University of Wisconsin
Madison, Wisconsin
United States

Chase Beal, DO
Department of Physical Medicine and Rehabilitation
    MetroHealth System/Case Western Reserve
    University
Cleveland, OH
United States

Brian R. Brenner, MD
Department of Anesthesiology
University of Virginia
Charlottesville, VA
United States

Ryan Budwany, MD, MPH, MBA
Director of Pain Medicine
CAMC Teays Valley Hospital
Spine and Nerve Centers of the Virginias
Hurricane, WV
United States

Ryan Steven D'Souza, MD
Pain Physician
Anesthesiology and Perioperative Medicine
Mayo Clinic Hospital
Rochester, MN USA

Jay Darji, DO
Temple University/Moss Rehabilitation
Philadelphia, PA
United States

Tyler Ericson, MD
Department of Anesthesiology
University of Virginia
Charlottesville, VA
United States

Steven M. Falowski, MD
Director Functional Neurosurgery
Neurosurgery
Neurosurgical Associates of Lancaster
Lancaster, PA
United States

Michael A. Fishman, MD, MBA
Interventional Pain Physician
Director of Research
Center for Interventional Pain and Spine
Lancaster, PA
United States

Mayank Gupta, MD
President and CEO
Kansas Pain Management and Neuroscience
    Research Center LLC
Overland Park, KS
Adjunct Clinical Assistant Professor
Kansas City University of Medicine and Biosciences
    President
Kansas Society of Interventional Pain Physicians
Kansas City, MO
United States

Michael Gyorfi, MD
Anesthesiology
University of Wisconsin School of Medicine and
    Public Health
Madison, WI
United States

Behnum Habibi, MD
Assistant Professor
Physical Medicine and Rehabilitation
Temple University Health System
Philadelphia, PA
United States

Jason Hamamoto, MD
Temple University/Moss Rehabilitation
Philadelphia, PA
United States

Chong Kim, MD
Professor
Department of Physical Medicine and Rehabilitation
MetroHealth System/Case Western Reserve University
    School of Medicine
Cleveland, OH
United States

Lynn Kohan, MD, MS
Professor of Anesthesiology and Pain Medicine
Department of Anesthesiology, Division of Pain
    Medicine
University of Virginia
Charlottesville, VA

Andrew Olsen, DO
Department of Physical Medicine and Rehabilitation
MetroHealth System/Case Western Reserve University
    School of Medicine
Cleveland, Ohio
United States

Priyanka Singla, MBBS, MD
Pain Medicine
Division of pain medicine
Department of Anesthesiology
University of Virginia
Charlottesville, VA
United States

Omar Viswanath, MD
Interventional Pain Medicine Physician,
    Anesthesiologist
Innovative Pain and Wellness
AZ;
Department of Anesthesiology, Creighton University
    School of Medicine
Omaha, NE;
Department of Anesthesiology, LSU Health
    Shreveport
Shreveport, LA
United States

Preface

Minimally invasive spinal fusion procedures are an evolving modality for treating chronic pain. Importantly, the development of percutaneous fusion devices and techniques has made it feasible for the pain physician to safely perform these procedures. However, prior to performing these procedures, knowledge of neuroaxial anatomy, an understanding of the indications and contraindications, sound procedural technique, and an ability to identify and manage any potential complications is needed.

To further assist the pain physician in adopting these techniques into their practice, we authored this book to provide a detailed guide on currently known minimally invasive spinal fusion procedures. In each chapter we highlight important anatomic considerations, aspects for patient selection, perioperative considerations, and procedural techniques with images for various minimally invasive spinal fusion procedures.

In developing this book, I would first like to thank my fellow coauthors who spent countless hours in curating information and contributing to this initiative. I would also like to thank my family who continues to support me in my research endeavors. Finally, I would like to thank the publisher, who has provided me and my fellow coauthors with many opportunities to contribute to the medical literature.

To close, I encourage the pain physician who is interested in learning more about, and potentially performing, minimally invasive spinal fusion procedures to use this book as a guide to supplement their practical learning. Learning new procedures can certainly be challenging, but I hope that with increasing knowledge you may consider minimally invasive spinal fusion procedures as part of your toolbox in treating patients with chronic pain.

Alaa Abd-Elsayed, MD, MPH, CPE, FASA

Contents

Chapter 1

Anatomy of Vertebrae

Andrew Olsen, Chase Beal, and Chong Kim

Introduction

The spine consists of 33 vertebrae: 24 presacral, 5 fused sacral, and 4 coccygeal. This structure together with the skull and the pelvis makes up the axial skeleton, which acts as the central column of rigid support and muscular/ligamentous attachment for the body. Of the 24 presacral vertebrae, 7 are in the cervical region between the head and ribs, 12 are thoracic, supporting the rib cage, and 5 are lumbar between the ribs and the sacrum. From the superior-most cervical vertebra (C1) to the inferior-most lumbar vertebra (L5), the vertebrae increase in size and mass to support the increasing load of the body and spinal column above (Fig. 1.1).[1]

Generally, with some differences applying between levels of the spine, vertebrae all have shared structures (Fig. 1.2). The vertebral body is the anterior-most section of each vertebra and is the primary load-bearing portion of the spinal column. Posterior to the vertebral body is the vertebral arch, which projects from the lateral aspects of the body. The pedicle is the portion of the arch attached to the body, while the lamina project from each pedicle to meet, completing the arch. From this point, the spinous process projects posteriorly. Situated on each pedicle are the superior and inferior articular processes, which articulate with the processes of the segment above and below forming the zygapophyseal joints (Z-joints) and the neural foramina. The transverse processes extend laterally from the pedicle and differ significantly from region to region, as will be highlighted later in this chapter. Aside from the structural support of the skeleton and muscular attachments, the spinal cord also protects the spinal cord, which passes through the spinal canal, a channel bound by the vertebral body anteriorly, and the vertebral arch posteriorly.[2]

CURVATURES

There are four curvatures in the adult spine—cervical, thoracic, lumbar, and sacral—with alternating convexity (Fig. 1.3). The cervical and lumbar curvatures are oriented with posterior concavity, known as lordosis, while the thoracic and sacral curvatures are oriented with anterior concavity, known as kyphosis.[3] The curvatures of the vertebral column change through development, from the developing fetus to adulthood. The fetal spine is anteriorly concave through its entire length (Fig. 1.4). In adulthood, the sacrum and the thoracic curvatures retain this anterior orientation, while the cervical and lumbar curvatures reverse, making them primary and secondary curvatures, respectively.

INTERVERTEBRAL DISC

Between each vertebral body is a fibrocartilaginous disc aptly named the intervertebral disc. These structures have three parts. These include the annulus fibrosus, a meshwork of interlocking collagen fibers, and other structural proteins wrapping in alternating orientation around the nucleus pulposus allowing it to withstand multidirectional stress. The nucleus is a gel-like center of the disc that is held tightly by the annulus fibrosis. It is over 80% water—making it noncompressible—which allows it to act as a shock absorber. The nucleus is made of up a loose network of collagen, proteoglycan, and elastin. Sandwiching these are the endplates of the intervertebral disc, which are the surfaces that articulate with the vertebrae above and below.

The intervertebral discs are poorly vascularized, relying on the diffusion of nutrients from adjacent vertebrae.[4] The innervation of the intervertebral discs is from the ventral rami and grey ramus communicans of the spinal nerves at the level above, so the L4-L5

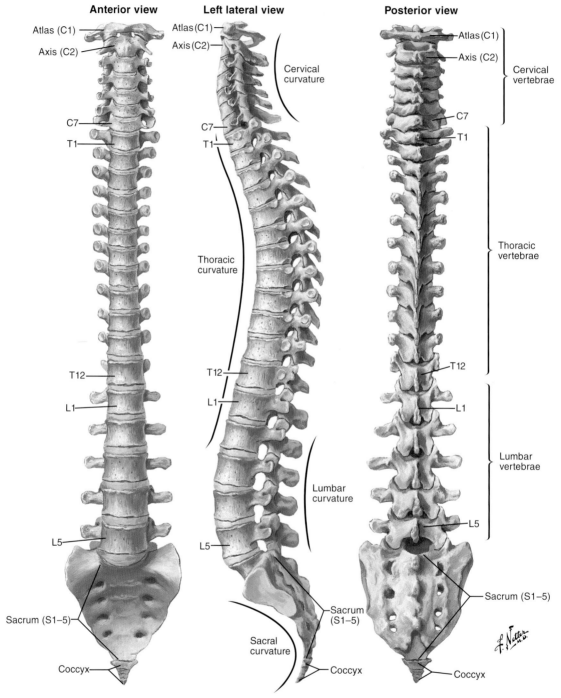

Anterior view

Atlas (C1)
Axis (C2)

C7
T1

T12

L1

L5

Sacrum (S1–5)

Coccyx

Left lateral view

Atlas (C1)
Axis (C2)

Cervical
curvature

C7
T1

Thoracic
curvature

T12
L1

Lumbar
curvature

L5

Sacrum
(S1–5)

Sacral
curvature

Coccyx

Posterior view

Atlas (C1)

Axis (C2)

Cervical
vertebrae

C7
T1

Thoracic
vertebrae

T12

L1

Lumbar
vertebrae

L5

Sacrum (S1–5)

Coccyx

Fig. 1.1 Anterior, lateral, and posterior views of the spinal column. This figure clearly shows the gradual increase in size from cervical to lumbar vertebrae as well as the curvatures of the spine as it transitions from cervical lordosis to thoracic kyphosis to lumbar lordosis and finally sacral and coccygeal kyphosis. (From Netter FH. *Atlas of Human Anatomy*. 5th ed. Saunders/Elsevier; 2010.)

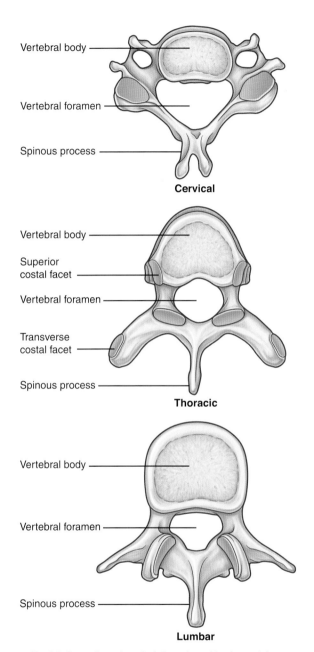

Vertebral body

Vertebral foramen

Spinous process

Cervical

Vertebral body

Superior
costal facet

Vertebral foramen

Transverse
costal facet

Spinous process

Thoracic

Vertebral body

Vertebral foramen

Spinous process

Lumbar

Fig. 1.2 Comparison of cervical, thoracic, and lumbar vertebrae.

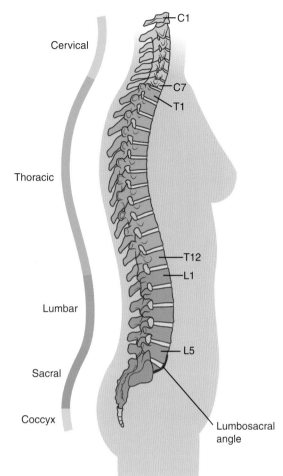

Cervical

C1

C7

T1

Thoracic

T12

L1

Lumbar

L5

Sacral

Coccyx

Lumbosacral
angle

Fig. 1.3 Curvatures of the adult spine.

disc is innervated by L4 (Fig. 1.5).[5] Attached to this bony framework are ligaments, tendons, deep, intermediate, and superficial muscles, which will be expanded upon later in this chapter. When combined with these connective structures, the spine can move in flexion and extension, right and left side bending, and can rotate around the central axis. The segments of the vertebrae articulate with each other at Z-joints. From top to bottom, cervical to lumbar, the superior articular surface of the facet joints of the vertebrae shift from being primarily upward and posterior facing in the cervical vertebrae to lateral and posterior facing in the thoracic vertebrae and finally medial and posterior in the lumbar. This is a gradual transition from level to level, and the shift in orientation allows for different freedom of movement for each region of the spine. The lumbar and cervical spine are both able to side bend and rotate to a similar degree. The cervical spine has the largest range of

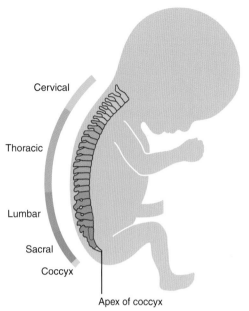

Cervical

Thoracic

Lumbar

Sacral

Coccyx

Apex of coccyx

Fig. 1.4 Curvature of the fetal spine.

motion in flexion, whereas the lumbar spine is most free in extension.[6] The thoracic spine, locked in place due to the attachment of the thoracic cage, is the freest in axial rotation.[7] The orientation of the facet joints can be best illustrated in Figs. 1.6 and 1.7.

ZYGAPOPHYSEAL JOINT

The (Z-Joints) are true joints made up of articular surfaces, a synovial membrane, and a joint capsule. They are innervated by the dorsal rami of spinal nerves. Two pairs of medial branch nerves from the dorsal rami, one from the level above and one below, join to provide innervation to the joint. By naming convention this means at the cervical level these two medial branches come from the same corresponding nerve level, so C5-C6 Z-joints are innervated by C5 and C6 medial branch nerves. Alternatively in the thoracic and lumbar regions due to the existence of the C8 to T1 transition the level of innervation is shifted, meaning that the T11-T12 facet joint

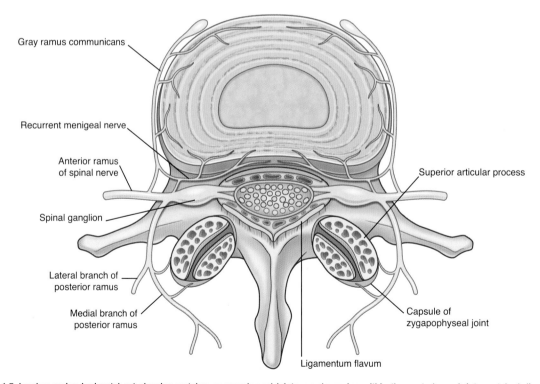

Gray ramus communicans

Recurrent menigeal nerve

Anterior ramus of spinal nerve

Spinal ganglion

Lateral branch of posterior ramus

Medial branch of posterior ramus

Superior articular process

Capsule of zygapophyseal joint

Ligamentum flavum

Fig. 1.5 Lumbar region horizontal cut showing vertebra, zygapophyseal joints, cauda equina within the central canal, intervertebral disc with innervations showing course of medial branches, gray ramus, recurrent meningeal, and penetration of the sinuvertebral nerves.

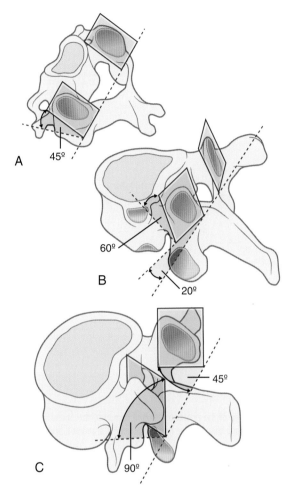

Fig. 1.6 3D depiction of the angle of orientation of the zygapophyseal joints of the (A) cervical, (B) thoracic, and (C) lumbar vertebrae.

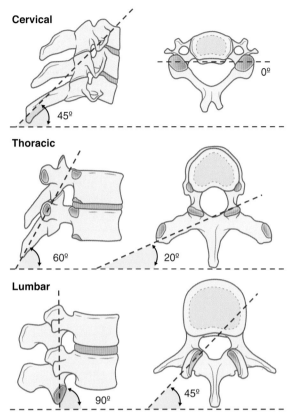

Fig. 1.7 2D representation of the orientation of the superior articular process at cervical, thoracic, and lumbar levels.

is innervated by T10 and T11 medial branches.[3] The course of the posterior ramus of the spinal nerves can be seen in Fig. 1.8.

NERVOUS SYSTEM

The nervous system of the spine is split between the central nervous system in the form of the spinal cord and the peripheral nervous system. As mentioned previously, the spine functions not only as rigid support and attachment for the body but also as a protective conduit for the spinal cord. The spinal cord is cylindrical in shape extends out from the skull via the foramen magnum and extends to roughly two-thirds the length

of the spine. Spinal cord is contained inside the dural sack with denticulate ligaments anchoring the cord to the dura between nerve roots. Inside the dural sack anterior and posterior to the denticulate ligaments are the anterior and posterior nerve rootlets, which meet to form the spinal nerves. The dura, the arachnoid, and the pia mater make up the meninges. The pia mater is the tissue layer sitting directly on top the spinal cord, whereas the arachnoid is between the pia mater and the dural sac.[3] The cord is bathed in cerebrospinal fluid, which is contained within the dural sac and below the arachnoid mater within the subarachnoid space (Fig. 1.9).

The spinal cord itself can be divided into white matter and grey matter, with the grey matter made up of cell bodies and the white matter made up of nerve tracts. The grey matter runs in a butterfly-shaped core through the center of the cord with white matter

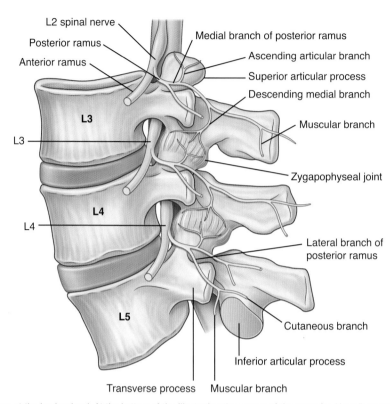

L2 spinal nerve
Posterior ramus
Anterior ramus
Medial branch of posterior ramus
Ascending articular branch
Superior articular process
Descending medial branch
Muscular branch
L3
L3
Zygapophyseal joint
L4
L4
Lateral branch of posterior ramus
L5
Cutaneous branch
Inferior articular process
Transverse process   Muscular branch

Fig. 1.8 The innervations at the lumbar level. At the bottom of the illustration the course of the posterior (dorsal) ramus of the spinal nerve can been seen coursing off the spinal nerve root, splitting into the medial and lateral branches then further into the articular branched, and muscular and cutaneous branches.

surrounding it. The spinal cord has anterior and posterior horns. The sensory function of the body arises in the posterior horn, whereas the motor function of the body arises from the anterior, making up the somatic nervous system.

The spinal nerves exit the spinal cord through neural foramina (visualized well in Fig. 1.8). From there, the nerves go on to innervate structures throughout the body. The sensory distribution of the spinal nerve levels is clearly mapped out in the dermatomes[1] (Fig. 1.10).

Cervical Spine

The cervical spine is made up of seven vertebrae, C1 to C7, descending from the skull towards the ribcage. The adult alignment of the cervical spine is lordotic in orientation.

BONES

C3 to C7 are what is referred to as "typical." This means that each possesses five shared features (Table 1.1). As alluded to previously, the vertebral body of C3 is the smallest in the human body and the vertebral bodies increase in size gradually (Figs. 1.11 and 1.12). The transverse processes of the cervical vertebrae are bifid, with anterior tubercles and posterior tubercles and the groove for the spinal nerve between (Fig. 1.13). Additionally, the vertebral artery courses through the foramen transversarium from C1 to C6.[8] Also bifid at the cervical level are the spinous processes (Fig. 1.12).

The Atypical Vertebrae

C1 (Atlas): The atlas is ring-shaped without either a vertebral body or spinous process. The ring is made of

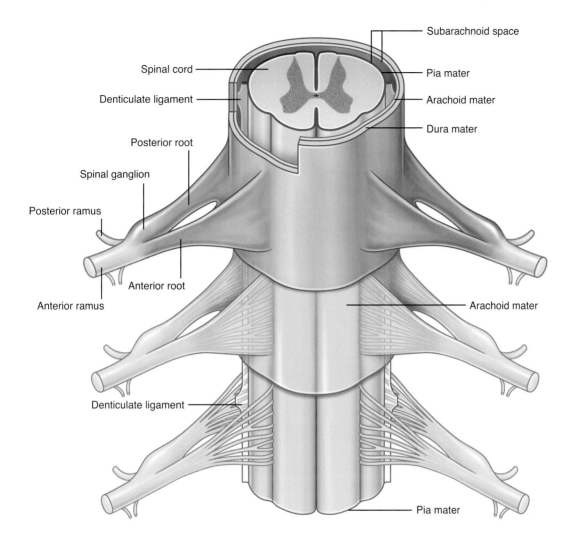

Fig. 1.9 Spinal cord and the meninges depicting the cord, denticulate ligament, pia, arachnoid, and dura mater, as well as the nerve rootlets and nerve roots.

two masses connected by arches anteriorly and posteriorly. On each of the lateral masses are the articular facets for articulation with adjacent vertebrae above and below. The superior facets of the atlas are concave in shape and articulate with the occiput, forming the atlanto-occipital joint. Posterior to each superior facet runs the groove for the vertebral artery. The inferior facets on the underside of the vertebra form the atlanto-axial joint. The ring is split by the transverse ligament of the atlas, which separates the dens of the axis anteriorly, from the spinal cord posteriorly (Fig. 1.14).

C2 (Axis): The axis has both a vertebral body and a spinous process. The feature that makes it distinct is the dens (odontoid process), which projects up from the vertebral body to articulate with the posterior aspect of the anterior arch of C1. This allows for free rotation of the skull (Figs. 1.15 and 1.16).

Ligaments

Ligaments of the cervical spine are discussed in this section, with some additions of universal ligaments across the spinal column. Structures are noted anteriorly to

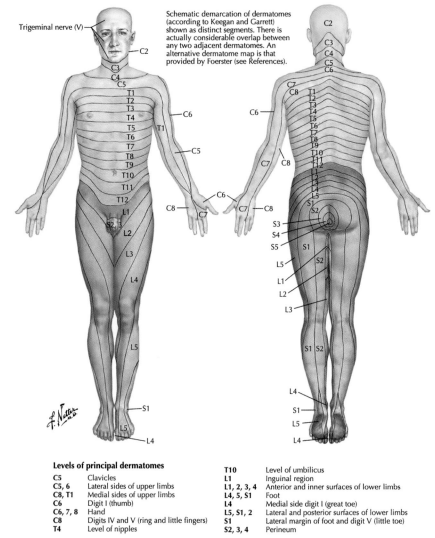

Schematic demarcation of dermatomes (according to Keegan and Garrett) shown as distinct segments. There is actually considerable overlap between any two adjacent dermatomes. An alternative dermatome map is that provided by Foerster (see References).

Levels of principal dermatomes

C5	Clavicles	T10	Level of umbilicus
C5, 6	Lateral sides of upper limbs	L1	Inguinal region
C8, T1	Medial sides of upper limbs	L1, 2, 3, 4	Anterior and inner surfaces of lower limbs
C6	Digit I (thumb)	L4, 5, S1	Foot
C6, 7, 8	Hand	L4	Medial side digit I (great toe)
C8	Digits IV and V (ring and little fingers)	L5, S1, 2	Lateral and posterior surfaces of lower limbs
T4	Level of nipples	S1	Lateral margin of foot and digit V (little toe)
		S2, 3, 4	Perineum

Fig. 1.10 Dermatomal distribution. (From Netter FH Atlas of Human Anatomy. Philadelphia: Saunders/Elsevier; 2014:162. 6th ed.)

TABLE 1.1 Bony Structures of the Cervical Spine

Structure	Description
Vertebral body	At the cervical level the structure is cupped superiorly with lateral uncinate processes locking into convex shape of the inferior portion of the vertebrae above. The anterior posterior dimension is shorter than the lateral dimension, making the cervical vertebra body oblong side to side.
Vertebral foramen	There is a large central foramen triangular in shape at the cervical level. The spinal cord passes through this foramen.
Transverse processes	Flat and lateral bodies at the cervical level function as muscular and ligamentous attachments and additionally house the transverse foramen.
Transverse foramen	Act as a conduit to allow for the vertebral arteries to pass on either side of the vertebral body. These are not present at C7.
Articular process	Point of articulation between vertebrae superiorly and inferiorly. At the cervical level superior articular processes are oriented superior posteriorly, whereas inferior articular processes are oriented anterior inferiorly.

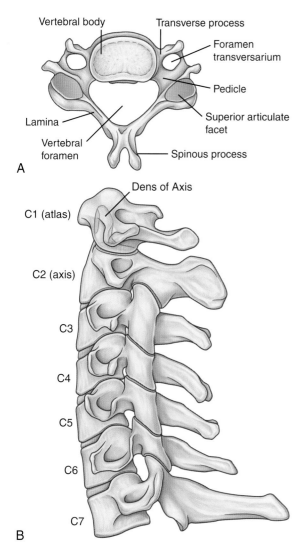

Fig. 1.11 Superior view (A) of one of the typical cervical vertebra C3 to C6, with a lateral view (B) of the cervical spine. Vertebral body; transverse process; foramen transversarium; pedicle; lamina; dens of axis; sinus processes of C2 and C3.

acts as a primary stabilizer of the spine limiting extension (Fig. 1.17, at the cervical level).

Apical ligament of the dens—This runs between the dens and the base of the skull and acts in the stabilization of the superior tip of the dens (Fig. 1.19).

Cruciform ligament—This is made up of the transverse ligament of the atlas and the superior and inferior longitudinal bands, which span from the axis to the skull base.[9] Acts in stabilization of the atlanto-axial joint, holding the dens against the articular cavity of the atlas, and anterior to the spinal cord (Figs. 1.14, 1.18, and 1.19).

*Posterior longitudinal ligament—This structure runs along the posterior aspect of the vertebral bodies from the base of the skull to the sacrum. Narrower than the anterior longitudinal ligament, limits the spine in flexion.

*Ligamentum flava (yellow ligament)—These ligaments exist throughout the spinal column and run between the laminae of adjacent vertebrae (Fig. 1.20).

*Interspinous ligament—Present throughout the spine, runs between adjacent spinous processes of vertebrae.

Nuchal ligament and supraspinous ligament— These are contiguous structures that extend from the occipital protuberance and median nuchal line on the skull to the spinous process of C7. Fibers of the nuchal ligament connect to the spinous processes of C2 to C7, and separate the cervical muscles R and L. Functions to limit flexion of the neck.

Muscles

The musculature of the cervical spine is in part shared with the thoracic spine with primary extensors passing the threshold from C7 to T1. The muscles of the atlanto-occipital junction must be mentioned for completeness.[10] They can be visualized in Fig. 1.21 and are listed with innervation, insertions, and actions in Table 1.2. The superficial movers of the shoulder girdle, namely trapezius, and levator scapulae are beyond the scope of this chapter.

Zygapophyseal Joint

The Z-joints of the cervical spine are oriented 45% upward and posterior with a neutral lateral angle.

posteriorly along the column. (* used to denote structures that extend beyond the cervical spine; Figs. 1.13 and 1.17–1.19.)

*Anterior longitudinal ligament—This broad ligament runs along the entirety of the spinal column from the base of the skull to the sacrum along the anterior aspect of the vertebral bodies of the cervical, thoracic, then lumbar spine. It

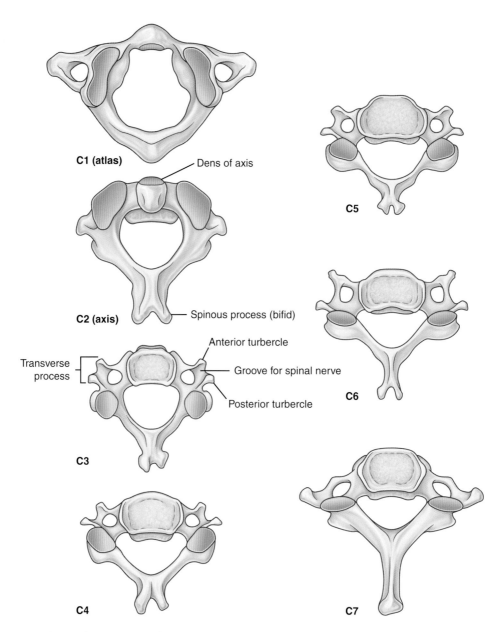

Fig. 1.12 Cervical vertebrae C1 to C7 clearly showing foramen transversarium and bifid spinous processes.

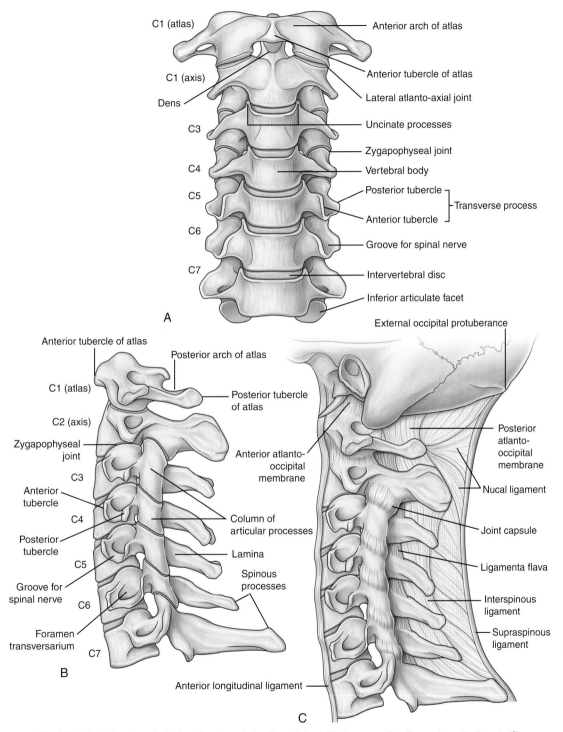

Fig. 1.13 Articulation of cervical spine, showing anterior (A) and lateral (B) views as well as ligamentous attachments (C).

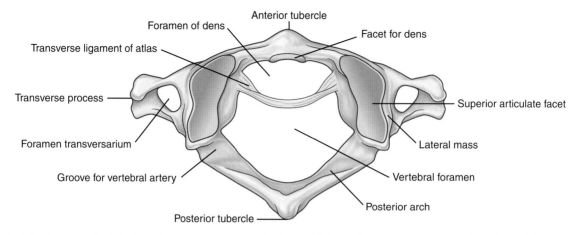

Fig. 1.14 C1 vertebra, the "atlas," seen from above with named structures labeled. Note the foramen for the dens where C2 articulates with C1 anteriorly.

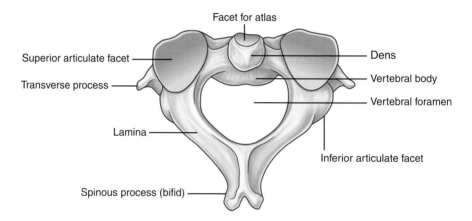

Fig. 1.15 C2 vertebra, the "axis," seen from above with named structures labeled.

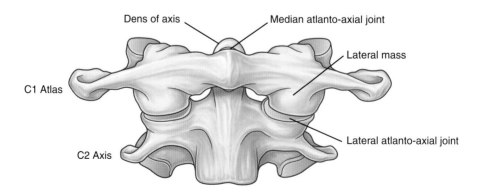

Fig. 1.16 Anterior view of C1-C2 articulation showing the dens of the axis as well as the Z-joints on the lateral masses.

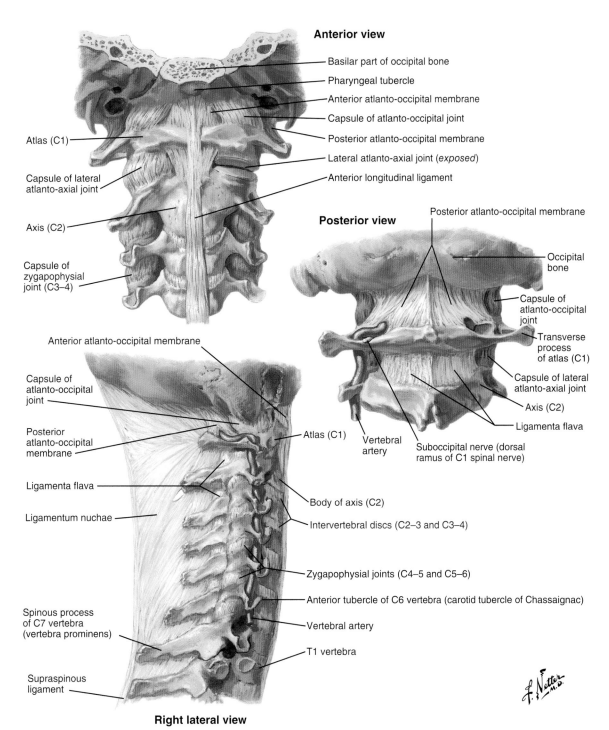

Anterior view

- Basilar part of occipital bone
- Pharyngeal tubercle
- Anterior atlanto-occipital membrane
- Capsule of atlanto-occipital joint
- Posterior atlanto-occipital membrane
- Lateral atlanto-axial joint (*exposed*)
- Anterior longitudinal ligament

Atlas (C1)

Capsule of lateral atlanto-axial joint

Axis (C2)

Capsule of zygapophysial joint (C3–4)

Posterior view

Posterior atlanto-occipital membrane

Occipital bone

Capsule of atlanto-occipital joint

Transverse process of atlas (C1)

Capsule of lateral atlanto-axial joint

Axis (C2)

Ligamenta flava

Anterior atlanto-occipital membrane

Capsule of atlanto-occipital joint

Posterior atlanto-occipital membrane

Ligamenta flava

Ligamentum nuchae

Atlas (C1)

Vertebral artery

Suboccipital nerve (dorsal ramus of C1 spinal nerve)

Body of axis (C2)

Intervertebral discs (C2–3 and C3–4)

Zygapophysial joints (C4–5 and C5–6)

Anterior tubercle of C6 vertebra (carotid tubercle of Chassaignac)

Vertebral artery

Spinous process of C7 vertebra (vertebra prominens)

T1 vertebra

Supraspinous ligament

Right lateral view

Fig. 1.17 The anterior longitudinal ligament seen from anterior view running longitudinally from skull base inferiorly can be seen in the *top left* image. The supraspinous ligament and nuchal ligament are noted in the *bottom left* image from a lateral view, and ligament lava is indicated from posterior and lateral viewpoint in the *right* and *left lower* images. (From Netter FH. *Atlas of Human Anatomy.* 5th ed. Saunders/Elsevier; 2010.)

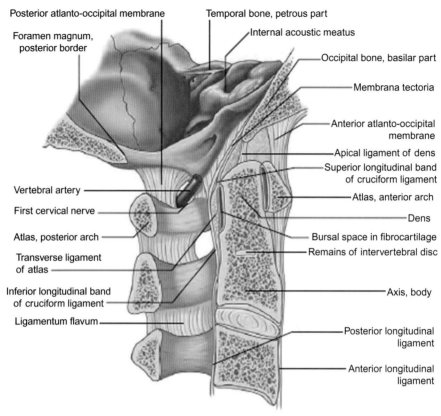

Posterior atlanto-occipital membrane

Foramen magnum, posterior border

Temporal bone, petrous part

Internal acoustic meatus

Occipital bone, basilar part

Membrana tectoria

Anterior atlanto-occipital membrane

Apical ligament of dens

Superior longitudinal band of cruciform ligament

Vertebral artery

First cervical nerve

Atlas, anterior arch

Dens

Atlas, posterior arch

Transverse ligament of atlas

Bursal space in fibrocartilage

Remains of intervertebral disc

Inferior longitudinal band of cruciform ligament

Ligamentum flavum

Axis, body

Posterior longitudinal ligament

Anterior longitudinal ligament

Fig. 1.18 Sagittal cut showing atlanto-axial-occipital joint. (From Angin Şimşek IE. *Comparative Kinesiology of the Human Body*. Elsevier; 2020:303-314.)

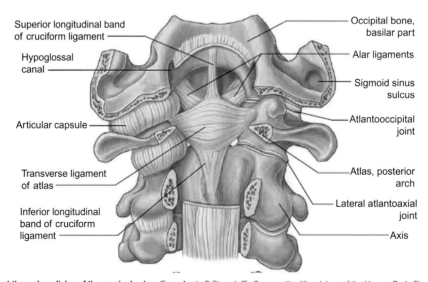

Superior longitudinal band of cruciform ligament

Hypoglossal canal

Articular capsule

Transverse ligament of atlas

Inferior longitudinal band of cruciform ligament

Occipital bone, basilar part

Alar ligaments

Sigmoid sinus sulcus

Atlantooccipital joint

Atlas, posterior arch

Lateral atlantoaxial joint

Axis

Fig. 1.19 Coronal cut through pedicles of the cervical spine. (From Angin S, Şimşek IE. *Comparative Kinesiology of the Human Body*. Elsevier; 2020:303-314.)

Left lateral view (*partially sectioned in median plane*)

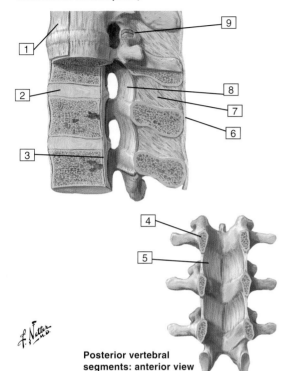

Posterior vertebral segments: anterior view

Fig. 1.20 Spinal *ligaments as demonstrated at the thoracic level.* *1,* Anterior longitudinal ligament; *2,* intervertebral disc; *3,* posterior longitudinal ligament; *4,* pedicle, transected; *5,* ligamentum flavum; *6,* supraspinous ligament; *7,* interspinous ligament; *8,* ligamentum flavum; *9,* zygapophyseal joint. (From Hansen JT, Netter F. Netter's Anatomy Flash Cards. 3rd ed. Philadelphia: Elsevier Health Sciences; 2012.)

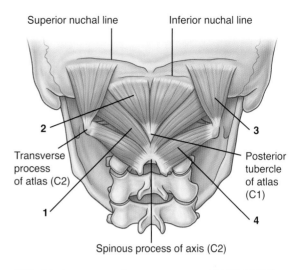

Superior nuchal line   Inferior nuchal line

Transverse process of atlas (C2)

Posterior tubercle of atlas (C1)

Spinous process of axis (C2)

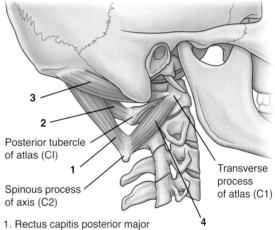

Posterior tubercle of atlas (CI)

Spinous process of axis (C2)

Transverse process of atlas (C1)

1. Rectus capitis posterior major
2. Rectus capitis posterior minor
3. Obliquus capitis superior
4. Obliquus capitis inferior

Fig. 1.21 The musculature at the junction of the cervical spine and the skull. Origins, insertions, actions, and innervations of muscles can be seen in Table 1.2.

They are innervated by the medial branches of the posterior rami of the spinal nerves at corresponding level.

Nervous System

The spinal cord at the cervical level is oval in shape and is the largest in size that it will be as it travels through the spine. The nerve roots that exit the spinal nerve at this level are numbered C1 to C8 and provide innervations to the phrenic nerve (C3, C4, C5), which innervates the diaphragm, and to the upper limbs. Adjacent to the spine anterolaterally course the sympathetic chain. At the cervical level this is in the form of the superior middle and inferior sympathetic cervical ganglia, supplying sympathetic innervation to structures in the head and neck.

Vasculature

The blood supply of the cervical spine is supplied by the vertebral and ascending vertebral arteries, which

TABLE 1.2	Muscles of Cervical Spine and Posterior Skull Base			
Muscle	Origin	Insertion	Innervation	Action
Rectus capitis posterior major	Spinous process of C2	Below the nuchal line on the lateral occipital bone	Posterior ramus of C1 spinal nerve	Extension and ipsilateral rotation of the skull
Rectus capitis posterior minor	Posterior tubercle of C1	Below nuchal line on medial occipital bone	Posterior ramus of C1 spinal nerve	Extension of the skull on atlas
Obliquus capitis superior	C1 transverse process	Between nuchal lines on occipital bone	Posterior ramus of C1 spinal nerve	Extension and ipsilateral side bending of skull
Obliquus capitis inferior	Spinous process of C2	Transverse process C1	Posterior ramus of C1 spinal nerve	Ipsilateral rotation of skull

arise from the subclavian and inferior thyroid arteries. The blood supply of the cervical spinal cord arises anteriorly from the anterior spinal artery, which descends from the vertebral arteries as they meet, as well as from the anterior segmental medullary arteries. Posteriorly the two posterior spinal arteries are fed by the posterior inferior cerebellar artery, as well as posterior segmental arteries off the vertebral arteries.

Thoracic Spine

The thoracic spine is defined by the articulation of the ribcage with the spine. There are 12 thoracic vertebrae numbered T1 to T12. They are anteriorly oriented with a kyphotic curve. Due to the semirigid attachments with the thoracic cage, the motion of the thoracic spine is limited in side-bending, flexion, and extension.

BONES

The vertebrae of the thoracic spine are all considered typical. At this level that means that each consists of the vertebral body, pedicle, lamina, transverse process, articular processes, and spinous process. Compared to the cervical vertebrae, which have rectangular vertebral bodies, the thoracic bodies are more heart shaped. Additionally, the transverse processes of the thoracic vertebrae are longer and project posterior laterally (Figs. 1.22 and 1.23).

MUSCLES

The intrinsic muscles of the thoracic level spine for the most part are shared in some degree or another with the cervical and lumbar regions. The deep layer of muscles

can be seen in Table 1.3. The intermediate layer of muscles of the back can been seen in Table 1.4.[11] The superficial layer of muscles of the thoracic region can be viewed in Table 1.5. Each of these listed muscles can be seen in Fig. 1.24. Large movers of the shoulder and upper extremities including trapezius, levator scapulae, rhomboid and latissimus dorsi, and the rotator cuff are beyond the scope of this chapter.

NERVOUS SYSTEM

Innervation of the thoracic spine includes the spinal cord and spinal nerves T1 to T12. Additionally, the sympathetic chain extends anterior lateral to the vertebral bodies sending sympathetic innervation to the organs of the thorax, abdomen, and pelvis.

VASCULATURE

The blood supply to the thoracic spine arises from the aorta via the posterior interosseous arteries (Fig. 1.25). The spinal cord also gets arterial supply from the spinal branches of the posterior intercostal arteries. Significantly, the anterior spinal artery anastomosis occurs at T9 with the artery of Adamkiewicz, which supplies the area distal to that level.[12]

Lumbar Spine

The lumbar spine consists of five vertebra levels extending from L1 with T12 above down to L5 with S1 below. They are neither bound by ribs nor the ala of the sacrum. The orientation of the adult lumbar spine is a natural lordosis.

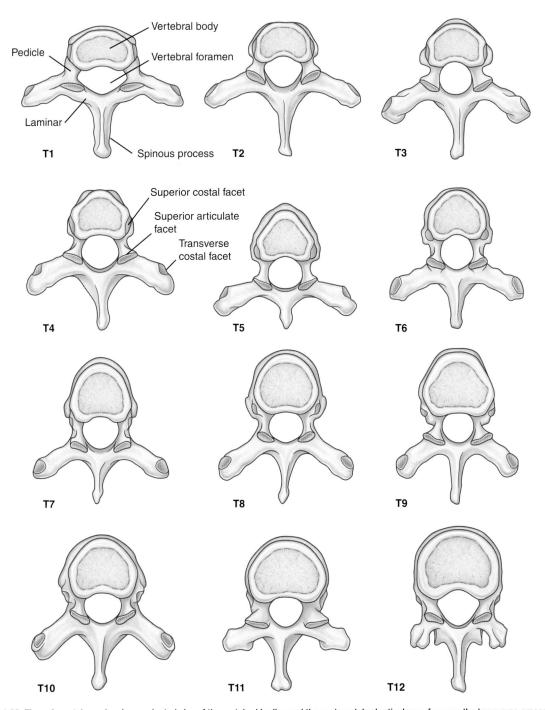

Fig. 1.22 Thoracic vertebrae showing graduated size of the vertebral bodies and the costovertebral articular surfaces on the transverse processes.

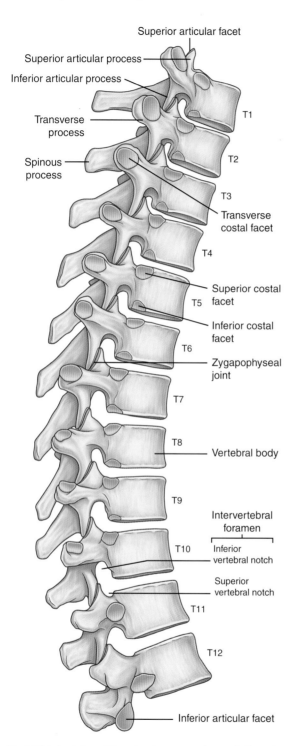

Superior articular facet

Superior articular process

Inferior articular process

Transverse process

Spinous process

T1

T2

T3

Transverse costal facet

T4

Superior costal facet

T5

Inferior costal facet

T6

Zygapophyseal joint

T7

T8   Vertebral body

T9

Intervertebral foramen

T10   Inferior vertebral notch

Superior vertebral notch

T11

T12

Inferior articular facet

Fig. 1.23 Lateral view of thoracic spine, curve not present. Shows increasing size of vertebral bodies going down the spine. Transition in the spinous process can also be seen in T10-T12 as it becomes shorter and less angled.

BONES

Lumbar vertebrae have the largest vertebral bodies as they accept and transfer the load of the entire body above them. Motion of the lumbar spine is free in flexion and extension as the orientation on the set joints is sagittal, with the inferior articular surfaces facing laterally and the superior articular surfaces facing medially (Figs. 1.26–1.28).

SOFT TISSUE

The ligaments of the lumbar region are largely unchanged from the major ligamentous structures listed earlier in this chapter. The anterior portion of the vertebral bodies is bound by the anterior longitudinal ligament, whereas the posterior aspect is linked by the posterior longitudinal ligament. The ligamentum flavum joints the adjacent laminae and between each spinous process runs the interspinous ligament. Along the posterior tip of the spinous processes runs the supraspinous ligament (Fig. 1.20).

NERVOUS SYSTEM

The spinal cord in the lumbar region ends at the conus medullaris, which ends at around L1 level in the adult spine. Below this level the filum terminal extends down to the coccyx and the spinal nerves to the lumbar and sacral regions continue in the cauda equina (Fig. 1.28).

VASCULATURE

The blood supply of the spinal cord in the lumbar region is supplied by the lumbar branches coming off the aorta.[3] Fig. 1.29 shows this at the level of T12 transitioning to the lumbar region, with lumbar artery coming off the aorta.

The spinal column, composed of 33 vertebrae, is an important part of the axial skeleton that provides rigid support while still allowing for motion in various planes. Although individual vertebrae may vary in shape, they typically share many common components and have the main function of protecting the spinal cord as it traverses caudally from the base of the skull. Each vertebrae communicates with those above and below through intervertebral discs, Z-joints, as well as various ligaments and muscle groups. This chapter describes the anatomy of the vertebrae and the unique elements found at the three main spinal levels: cervical, thoracic, and lumbar.

TABLE 1.3	Deep Intrinsic Muscles of the Back			
Muscle	**Superior Attachments**	**Interior Attachments**	**Innervation**	**Action**
Interspinalis	Inferior aspect of the spinous process, C and L spine	Superior aspect of the spinous process C and L spine	Posterior rami of spinal nerves	Extension and minor rotation of spine
Intertransversarii	Transverse processes of L and C vertebrae	Transverse process of L and C vertebrae	Posterior and anterior rami of spinal nerves	Lateral flexion of spine when acting unilaterally. Stabilization when acting bilaterally
Levatores costarum breves and longi	Transverse process C8-T11	Ribs between angle and tubercle	Posterior rami C8-T11 spinal nerves	Aid in elevation of the ribs for respiration
Semispinalis—divided into lumborum, thoracis, cervicis based on region	Attaches to Occiput and spinous processes of head and vertebrae 4–6 segments above origin	Originates from transverse processes of T and C vertebrae.	Posterior rami	Extension and contralateral rotation
Multifidi—divided into lumborum, thoracis, cervicis based on region	Attached to the spinous process of vertebra two to four segments superior	Sacrum, transverse processes of L2 through L5 and articular processes of C4 through C7	Posterior rami	Stabilization, primarily
Rotatores longest—thoracis and lumborum based on region	Originates junction of inferior aspect of lamina and spinous process of T and L vertebrae	Attaches to the transverse process a vertebra one to two segments below	Posterior rami	Local extension and rotation
Rotatores breves—thoracic and lumborum based on region	Originates at junction of inferior aspect of lamina and spinous process T and L vertebrae	Attaches to transverse process on vertebrae one segment below	Posterior rami	Local extension and rotation

TABLE 1.4	Intermediate Intrinsic Muscles of the Back			
Muscle	**Superior Attachment**	**Inferior Attachment**	**Innervation**	**Action**
Iliocostalis—cervicis, thoracic, lumbar based on region	Cervical transverse processes, Inferior aspect angles of ribs	Originates posterior portion of iliac crest, posterior surface of the sacrum, sacral and inferior lumbar spinous processes and supraspinous ligament	Posterior rami	Lateral bend when acting unilaterally, extension when acting bilaterally
Longissimus—cervicis, thoracic, lumbar based on region	Inferior aspect of ribs between angle and tubercle, into the mastoid process	Originates posterior portion of iliac crest, posterior surface of the sacrum, sacral and inferior lumbar spinous processes and supraspinous ligament	Posterior rami	Lateral bending when acting unilaterally, extension when acting bilaterally
Spinalis—cervicis, thoracic, lumbar based on region	Spinous processes of upper thoracic and the skull	Originates posterior portion of iliac crest, posterior surface of the sacrum, sacral and inferior lumbar spinous processes and supraspinous ligament	Posterior rami	Lateral bending when acting unilaterally, extension when acting bilaterally

TABLE 1.5	Superficial Intrinsic Muscles of the Back			
Muscle	**Superior Attachment**	**Inferior Attachment**	**Innervation**	**Action**
Splenius capitis	Lateral third of the nuchal line of the occiput and mastoid process	Spinous process and nuchal ligament of C7 through T6	Posterior rami	Lateral side bend and ipsilateral rotation when acting unilaterally, extend when acting bilaterally
Splenius cervicis	Transverse processes and posterior tubercles of C1 through C4	Spinous process and nuchal ligament of C7 through T6	Posterior rami	Ipsilateral rotation when acting unilaterally, extend when acting bilaterally

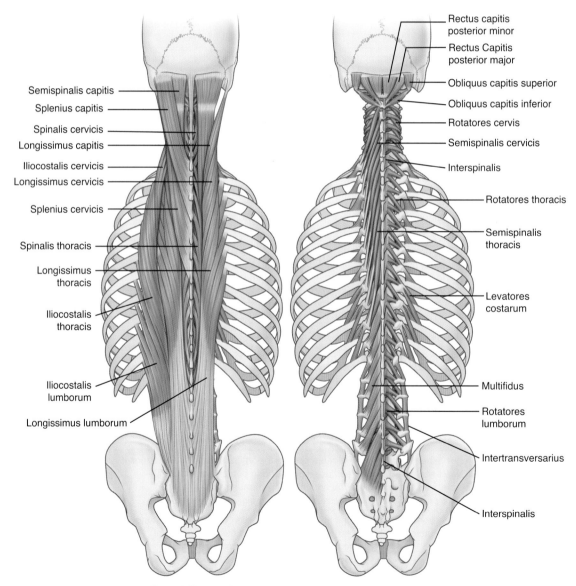

Fig. 1.24 The deep, intermediate, and superficial muscles of the spine.

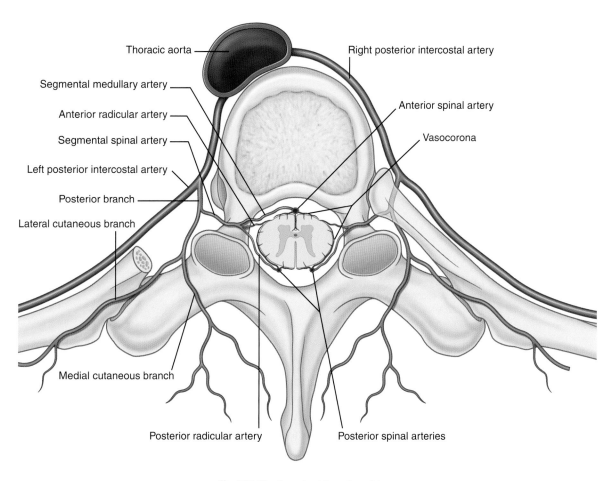

Fig. 1.25 Blood supply of thoracic vertebrae.

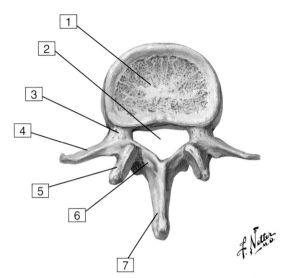

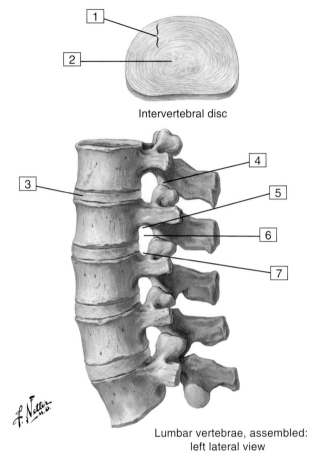

Intervertebral disc

Lumbar vertebrae, assembled:
left lateral view

Fig. 1.26 Lumbar vertebra. *1*, Large oval vertebral body; *2*, spinal canal; *3*, pedicle; *4*, transverse process; *5*, superior articular process; *6*, lamina; *7*, spinous process. *(From Hansen JT, Netter F. Netter's Anatomy Flash Cards. 3rd ed. Philadelphia: Elsevier Health Sciences; 2012.)*

Fig. 1.27 Bones and intervertebral disc *demonstrated at Lumbar level:* *1*, Annulus fibrosus; *2*, nucleus pulposus; *3*, intervertebral disc; *4*, zygapophyseal joint; *5*, inferior vertebral notch; *6*, neural foramen; *7*, superior vertebral notch. *(From Hansen JT, Netter F. Netter's Anatomy Flash Cards. 3rd ed. Philadelphia: Elsevier Health Sciences; 2012.)*

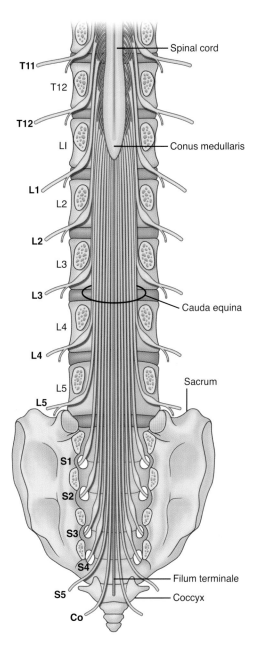

Fig. 1.28 The spine from T10 to coccyx with spinal cord, conus medullaris and caudal equina, filum terminal, and associated structures exposed.

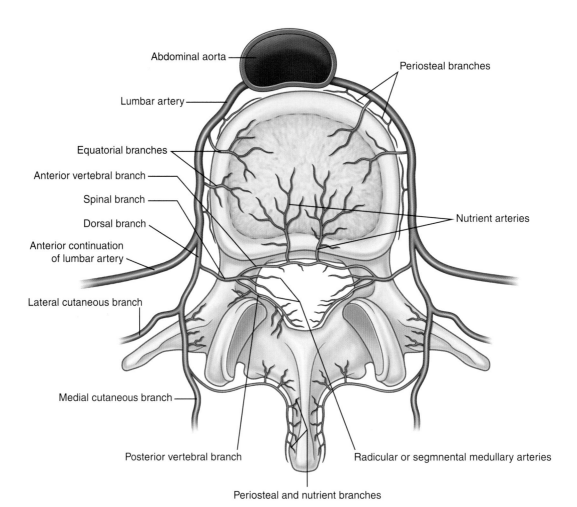

Abdominal aorta

Periosteal branches

Lumbar artery

Equatorial branches

Anterior vertebral branch

Spinal branch

Dorsal branch

Anterior continuation of lumbar artery

Nutrient arteries

Lateral cutaneous branch

Medial cutaneous branch

Posterior vertebral branch

Radicular or segmnental medullary arteries

Periosteal and nutrient branches

Fig. 1.29 The arterial supply and anatomy of the spine seen at the thoracic level. Named arterial branches are labeled.

REFERENCES

1. Netter FH. *Atlas of Human Anatomy*. 5th ed. Philadelphia: Saunders/Elsevier; 2010.
2. Tank PW. *Grant's Dissector*. 15th ed. Philadelphia: Lippincott Williams and Wilkins; 2013.
3. Moore KL, Agur AMR, Dalley AF II. *Essential Clinical Anatomy*. 5th ed. Philadelphia: Wolters Kluwer Health; 2015.
4. Frost BA, Camarero-Espinosa S, Foster EJ. Materials for the spine: anatomy, problems, and solutions. *Materials (Basel)*. 2019; 12(2):253.
5. Cramer G, Darby S, Frysztak R. *Pain of Spinal Origin*. Published June 11, 2016. Available at: https://basicmedicalkey.com/pain-of-spinal-origin-2/. Accessed July 26, 2021.
6. Gonzalez F, Dickman C. *Anatomy of the Spine and Spinal Cord*. Published February 8, 2017. Available at: https://neupsykey.com/anatomy-of-the-spine-and-spinal-cord-2/. Accessed July 26, 2021.
7. Poluyi T. *Control System Development for Six Degree of Freedom Spine Simulator*. Published August, 2014. Available at: https://www.researchgate.net/figure/Approximate-orientation-of-the-lower-cervical-A-thoracic-B-and-lumbar-C-facet_fig4_270340667. Accessed July 26, 2021.
8. Agur AMR, Dalley AF. *Grant's Atlas of Anatomy*. 13th ed. Philadelphia: Lippincott Williams and Wilkins; 2012.
9. Angin S, Şimşek IE Kinesiology of the cervical vertebral column. In: Akcali O, Satoglu IS, Cakiroglu MA, eds. *Comparative Kinesiology of the Human Body*. London, UK: Elsevier; 2020: 303–314.
10. Drake R, Vogl AW, Mitchell A. *Gray's Atlas of Anatomy and Gray's Anatomy for Students*. 2nd ed. Philadelphia: Churchill Livingstone; 2009.
11. Henson B, Kadiyala B, Edens MA. *Anatomy, Back, Muscles*. [Updated 2021 Aug 10]. In: StatPearls [Internet] Treasure Island (FL): StatPearls Publishing; 2022 https://www.ncbi.nlm.nih.gov/books/NBK537074/.
12. Amboss. *Vertebral column*. Accessed July 27, 2021. Available at: https://www.amboss.com/us/knowledge/Vertebral_column/.
13. Hansen JT, Netter F Netter's Anatomy Flash Cards. Philadelphia: Elsevier Health Sciences; 2012. 3rd ed.
14. Netter FH Atlas of Human Anatomy. Philadelphia: Saunders/Elsevier; 2014:162. 6th ed.

Chapter 2

Surgical Instruments

Brian R. Brenner, Tyler Ericson, Priyanka Singla, and Lynn Kohan

Common Instruments Used During Surgical Procedures of the Spine

In general, vertebrae get larger cranial to caudal; thus as a general rule of thumb instrument size for spine procedures increases in size from cervical (C) spine to lumbar (L) spine. The purpose of this chapter is to orient the proceduralist to common surgical equipment encountered for basic surgical skills.

Of note, specific tools for the accomplishment of various fusion procedures will not be covered in this chapter. The tools that are unique to the company-made kits will be further discussed in the chapters covering those specific procedures. We have grouped instruments according to their use.

Instruments Used for Making an Incision

SCALPELS

Scalpels are used for general skin incision. They have two parts—blade and handle. The belly of the blade is used for making the incision.

Scalpels come in various sizes, such as the #10 blade shown in Fig. 2.1. There are other-sized scalpel blades not referenced in this text.

Scalpels are very sharp instruments and cause injury if not handled appropriately. Safety precautions can prevent accidental laceration of the hand or body of the provider. Some of these include attaching the blade to the handle with the help of a forceps, marking the skin before incision, and holding the scalpel with the dominant hand. The scalpel is used to make superficial incisions through the epidermis and dermis partially into the subcutaneous tissue below.[1]

Countertraction of the skin, either with the operator's other hand or from an assistant, can be helpful in achieving a straight smooth cut in one motion.[1] A sharps safety tray (Fig. 2.2) should always be used to pass sharp instruments between the surgical field and the scrub nurse's Mayo stand. This aids in prevention of accidents and stick injuries with sharps and needles.[1] It is common courtesy to use clear language such as "sharp back," "passing sharp," "knife down," or "needle down and/or protected" when passing or moving instruments that have the potential to cause injuries.

BLADE SIZES

The #10 blade is the most commonly used blade for skin incisions. Fig. 2.1 shows a standard #10 blade with a #3 handle.

Instruments Used for Dissection

Once initial incision has been made with a scalpel, hemostasis is achieved with electrosurgical instruments. Dissection of tissues to adequately expose the structures of interest can be accomplished with electrosurgical, blunt, or sharp tools.

Electrosurgery

When an electrical current encounters a substance with resistance, heat is generated. Because all body tissue has an inherent resistance, this principle can be used to selectively cut, desiccate, fulgurate, or coagulate tissue. Electrosurgery is the utilization of a high-frequency alternating current to generate heat at a particular tissue for a desired surgical effect.[2]

TYPES OF ELECTROSURGERY

Electrosurgery can be either monopolar (Fig. 2.3), or bipolar (Fig. 2.4),[3] depending on the path the current takes.

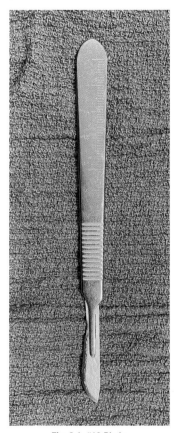

Fig. 2.1 #10 Blade.

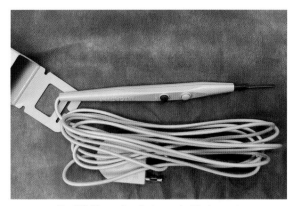

Fig. 2.3 Monopolar electrosurgical instrument.

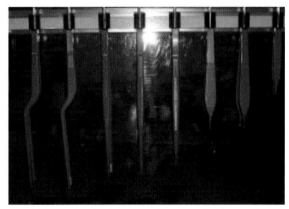

Fig. 2.4 Various bipolar electrosurgical instruments.[3] (Published with permission from Ustatine RP, Pfenninger JL, Stulberg DL, Small R. *Dermatologic and Cosmetic Procedures in Office Practice.* Elsevier; 2012.)

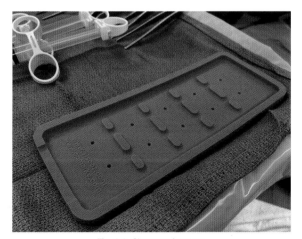

Fig. 2.2 Sharps safety tray.

In a *monopolar system*, there are two electrodes. One is the active surgical instrument and the other is a dispersion pad, which must be located far from the surgical site and have a large surface area. Inappropriate placement or inadequate surface area of the dispersion pad can result in severe burns.[4,5]

In a *bipolar system*, the electrical current flows between two electrodes, which are both located on the surgical instrument (forceps, scissors, graspers).

ADVANTAGE OF BIPOLAR ELECTROSURGERY

With a bipolar system there is less unintended heat spread. Bipolar electrosurgery is also better at providing hemostasis because the tissue is compressed between the two electrodes and then heated. A schematic

Bipolar and monopolar electrosurgery

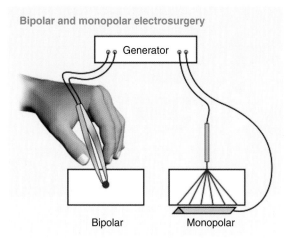

Fig. 2.5 General schematic of a monopolar versus bipolar electrosurgical systems.[2] (Published with permission from Hay DJ. Electrosurgery. *Surgery (Elsevier)*. 2007;26(2):66-69.)

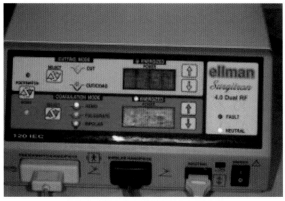

Fig. 2.6 Mono and bipolar wall unit illustrating cut versus coagulation controls that are common to many electrosurgical units.[3] (Published with permission from Ustatine RP, Pfenninger JL, Stulberg DL, Small R. *Dermatologic and Cosmetic Procedures in Office Practice*. Elsevier; 2012.)

of the dispersion of energy in a bipolar versus monopolar electrosurgical system is shown in Fig. 2.5

MODES OF ELECTROSURGERY

Electrocautery can be used in cut or coagulation mode. Current frequency, time of activation, and the use of continuous or intermittent waveforms can be changed to adjust the amount of heat generated during electrosurgery.

Cut mode uses a continuous, low-voltage current that forms a more concentrated area of high current density that results in a more rapid heating of tissue. The alternating current causes intense vibration and heat within the cells, causing them to vaporize, effectively cutting the tissue.[5] When using the cutting mode the electrode should be held close to the tissue, but not in direct contact. Despite being called cut mode, this mode is also effective at coagulation and generally results in less collateral thermal injury than coagulation mode.[6]

Coagulation mode utilizes an interrupted, high-voltage current over a larger surface area. Because the current is interrupted, the tissue has time to cool, resulting in coagulation rather than vaporization.[4] A downside of the higher voltage is more tissue damage and more thermal spread, increasing the risk of complications.

Because cutting mode is also effective at coagulation but with less risk of complications, many recommend only using coagulation mode when dealing with highly vascular tissue or tissue with poor conductivity such as adipose tissue. A common mono- and bipolar wall unit with corresponding cut versus coagulation functions is shown in Fig. 2.6.

COMPLICATIONS

Complications from the use of electrosurgery are relatively common, with approximately incidents 2 to 5 per 1000 procedures.[4,5] The most common adverse events are thermal burns and hemorrhage, with fire being a rare complication. The use of higher power settings with higher voltage causes more thermal spread and tissue damage. Severe burns can occur if the dispersion electrode pad becomes partially detached, minimizing the effective surface area and focusing the current on a smaller portion of the skin. In patients with electrical implants, it is ideal to use a bipolar device and to assess the function of the implant after surgery.

Tissue Dissection

Blunt dissection moves tissue planes without cutting, reducing bleeding risk and chance of incising important surrounding structures. Overly forceful blunt dissection should be limited to decrease chance of wound complications such as seroma formation, infection, and prolonged healing.

Sharp dissection results in less general tissue trauma at the cost of increased bleeding, which may be problematic. This can be mitigated by utilization of electrosurgical dissection in the cut mode.

Overall, some combination of gentle blunt, sharp, and electrosurgical dissection will need to be utilized to achieve the safe desired exposure.[1]

Scissors

Scissors are used for cutting and dissection of various tissues. They can be either sharp or blunt. The shape and size of this instrument is based on its intended function and purpose. A few commonly used scissors for interventional pain procedures are listed here. This is not a complete list and is intended to familiarize the reader with this class of instrument.

METZENBAUM SCISSORS

These scissors have a number of variations. They can have blunt or sharp tips and can either be curved or straight. Applications include blunt dissection of tissue or cutting of tissue for dissection. Metzenbaum scissors are smaller than the similar Mayo scissor (Fig. 2.7). The benefit is a more equal cutting and dissecting tip in relation to the length of the shaft, which gives the operator more finite control of the instrument in small or anatomically vulnerable areas. The disadvantage is smaller size and less force generation for cutting and dissecting of stronger tissue such as muscle or fascia.[1]

MAYO SCISSORS

Mayo scissors are similar in function to the Metzenbaum scissors but larger in size with a longer shaft to cutting tip ratio. They are better suited for larger areas of dissection where precise control is less important, as well as for cutting more robust tissue such as muscle or fascia (Fig. 2.8).[1]

Suction

Suction instruments are used for aspirating fluid such as blood, secretions, and saline from a wound or body orifice. The most commonly used globally is the

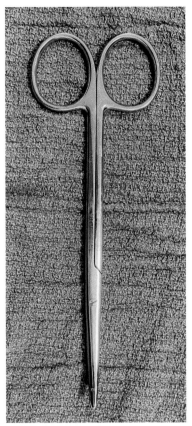

Fig. 2.7 Metzenbaum scissors.

Yankauer (Fig. 2.9), and there are smaller suction instruments for working in small, delicate anatomic areas. Suction often needs to be clamped with a tool such as an Allis clamp (see "Allis Clamp" section and Fig. 2.21) while not in use to turn "off" the suction.[1]

Yankauer—Usually made out of plastic or metal, this suction device was invented by otolaryngologist Sidney Yankauer in 1907 for use during tonsillectomies.[5] The Yankauer is now used for a variety of applications. It has a rigid, slightly angled tip that can be used for everything from oropharyngeal suction to blood evacuation from the surgical field during exposure and closure. Its bulbous tip enables delicate suction of structures without damaging surrounding tissue.

Instruments Used for Retraction

Retractors come in hundreds of shapes and sizes. The use of a particular retractor depends on surgeon

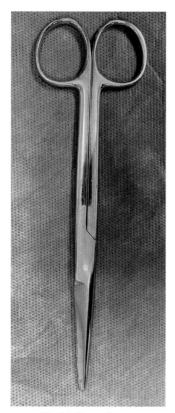

Fig. 2.8 Mayo scissors.

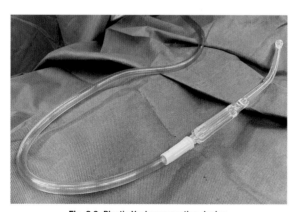

Fig. 2.9 Plastic Yankauer suction device.

preference, comfort, and familiarity. They can be self-retaining, large with prominent grips and lever arms, or small and thin for finite elevation and exposure of tissue. Some of the most common basic retractors for exposure are listed here with their functional advantages.[1]

WEITLANER RETRACTOR

This is used for superficial skin and muscle retraction. It is self-retaining; thus once initial exposure is achieved, the instrument will hold that position until released (Fig. 2.10).[1]

D'ERRICO RETRACTOR/CEREBELLAR RETRACTOR

This retractor is longer and thinner than the Weitlaner. It is similar in function to the Weitlaner but better suited for deeper and longer incisions (Fig. 2.11).[7]

MEYERDING RETRACTOR

This retractor is used for deeper incisions. It is similar in function to the previously mentioned retractors (Weitlaner, D'Errico) but with flat metal tips that are best suited for deep retraction. The edges are a single

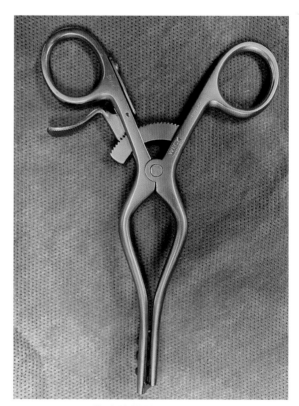

Fig. 2.10 Weitlaner retractor.

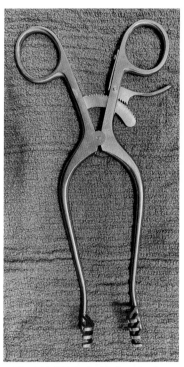

Fig. 2.11 D'Errico/cerebellar retractor.

unit of metal, as compared to the teeth-like design of the D'Errico (Fig. 2.12).[7]

RICHARDSON RETRACTOR

Often called a "Rich," this retractor comes in multiple shapes and sizes and is used to retract soft tissue during dissection. It is used for deeper retraction than other instruments in this category (Fig. 2.13).[8]

PHRENIC RETRACTOR

This is similar in function to the Rich, but has a light, hollow handle allowing for more finite control (Fig. 2.14).

ARMY-NAVY RETRACTOR

This is a double-sided retractor with one shallow and one deep side. It is used for retraction of soft tissue and structures in a similar fashion to the previously mentioned instruments (Rich, phrenic) (Fig. 2.15).

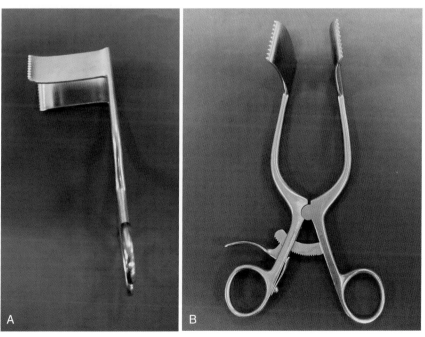

Fig. 2.12 Meyerding retractor. (A) Profile and (B) anterior view.

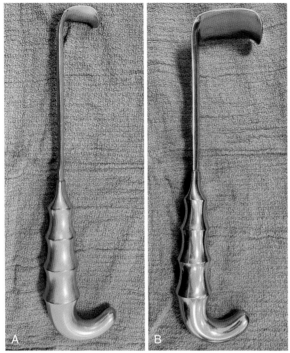

Fig. 2.13 Richardson ("rich") retractors of various sizes. (A) Small. (B) Large.

Elevators

Elevators are surgical tools that come in various shapes and sizes and are suited for lifting the periosteum off the bone for spine exposure. They are also adept at muscle retraction and elevation for further exposure of the spine.[7]

KEY ELEVATOR

This common elevator is used in interventional spine procedures for exposure of the various osteographic components of the spine (Fig. 2.16).

Instruments Used for Clamping or Grasping

FORCEPS/HEMOSTATS

Forceps is a term that comes from the Latin word *forca*, meaning snare or trap.[1] It is a term unique to medicine and is used to describe a class of surgical instruments that are either tweezers or clamps that rely on lever arms to grab, clamp, and secure various tissues, instruments, and surgical equipment. The main categories

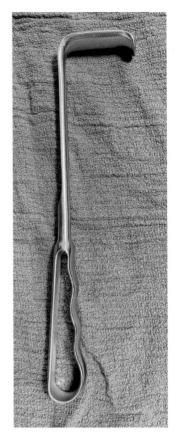

Fig. 2.14 Phrenic retractor.

are locking and nonlocking, and they are used for everything from hemostasis to closure. For the purpose of grouping instruments according to their use, the nonlocking forceps common in interventional pain procedures will be included in the "Closure" section.

Locking Forceps

SPONGE-STICK FORCEPS

A sponge-stick forceps is an instrument designed to clamp a surgical sponge to remove small amounts of fluid from the surgical field. It can also be used to tamponade and provide pressure to areas of bleeding in the surgical field (Fig. 2.17).

MAYO FORCEPS

The Mayo forceps has interlocking teeth that lock and provide constant pressure once engaged. It is used for

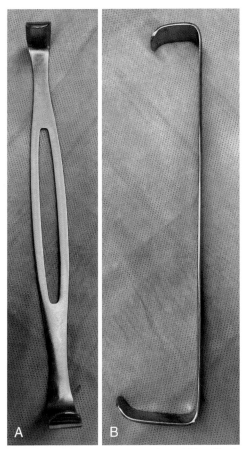

Fig. 2.15 Army-Navy retractor. (A) Anterior and (B) profile view.

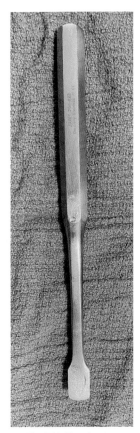

Fig. 2.16 Key elevator.

various applications in all phases of surgery, including hemostasis, exposure, dissection, and closure. Mayo forceps are large locking forceps second only in size to the tonsil forceps (Fig. 2.18).[1]

KELLY FORCEPS

The Kelly forceps performs the same function as the Mayo forceps, but is smaller in size (medium-sized interlocking forceps) (Fig. 2.19).

MOSQUITO FORCEPS

The smallest of the interlocking teeth forceps, these are better suited for working in anatomic locations that require small, precise movement. They are often used to clamp ties for blood vessel management, and they can also be used to tag sutures (Fig. 2.20).

ALLIS CLAMP

This is an interlocking forceps with sharp teeth at the bottom of the instrument used to hold and grasp tissue and fascia. It has a slightly rounded jaw (Fig. 2.21).[8]

KOCHER CLAMP

This traumatic straight-toothed clamp is used for holding heavy tissue and fascia, often when the tissue will be removed later (Fig. 2.22).[8]

Instruments and Materials for Wound Closure

Another part of the proceduralist's armamentarium are closure devices. They are too numerous to include all for the purpose of this text but include items such as suture needles, thread, ties, needle drivers, forceps, staples, surgical adhesives, gels,

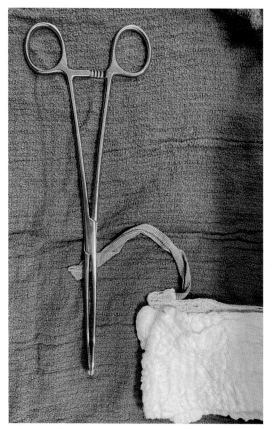

Fig. 2.17 Sponge-stick forceps alongside a surgical sponge.

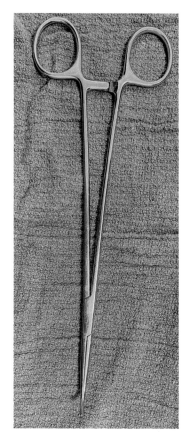

Fig. 2.18 Mayo clamp.

foams, and tension strips. This text will review common basic surgical closure devices and components used for simple wound closure most commonly encountered in the interventional pain setting. Closure device and tool choice will alter aspects such as healing time, cosmesis of the wound, and integrity of the regenerating tissue. Simple suture is the most frequently encountered and will be discussed in detail in the next section.[1]

Suture

The approximation of wound edges is critical to the healing of a surgical incision. This is commonly achieved using sutures of various types (Fig. 2.23). The particular type of suture varies largely on the material from which they are made. Suture type is selected according to the location of sutured tissue,

healing time of tissue, underlying strength of the tissue being sutured, and the desired absorption profile.

NATURAL VERSUS SYNTHETIC

Natural sutures can be made from cotton, sheep gut mucosa, beef serosa, or silk. Synthetic sutures include Dacron, nylon, polyester, and others. An advantage is that they do not produce as intense an inflammatory reaction as natural sutures.

ABSORPTION PROFILE

Absorbable sutures are made of either mammalian collagen or synthetic polymers that undergo hydrolysis or enzymatic breakdown after a specific period of time. They are often used for deep layers of tissue that would be harder to access for later removal. Nonabsorbable sutures are made from synthetic materials like nylon or polypropylene and require removal after

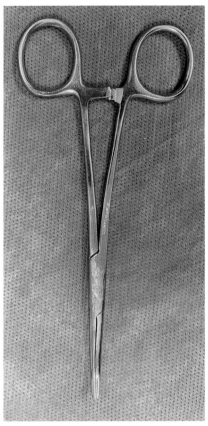

Fig. 2.19 Kelly clamp.

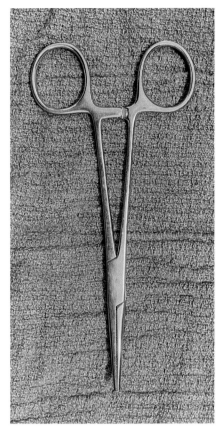

Fig. 2.20 Mosquito clamp.

placement. Nonabsorbable sutures become surrounded by fibrotic tissue but have the advantages of being easier to handle and able to stretch to allow for wound swelling.

MONOFILAMENT VERSUS MULTIFILAMENT

Monofilament sutures consist of many fibers that run in parallel and are not braided or twisted. Benefits of monofilament sutures are that they do not traumatize the tissue as much as multifilament sutures do and they resist harboring microorganisms; both reasons making them better for subcuticular closure.[9] Disadvantages are that they require more knots than multifilament and can stretch up to 30% before breaking, making them suboptimal for deep layers.

Multifilament sutures consist of multiple fibers braided together. They are easier to handle and tie and have more stable knots than monofilament sutures.

SUTURE SIZE

Suture sizing commonly uses the United States Pharmacopeia (USP) system in which the number preceding zero inversely correlates with size. For instance a 3-0 suture would be larger than a 6-0. Generally, larger sutures are associated with greater inflammation and scarring. A commonly used suture scheme would be 2-0 or 3-0 absorbable and braided suture such as Vicryl (Fig. 2.23B,C) for the closure of deep layers, and a 4-0 absorbable monofilament suture such as Monocryl (Fig. 2.23D,E) for superficial layers.

Adhesives

Although sutures are the common closure method of choice because of their high tensile strength and low failure rate, a drawback is that suturing requires the traumatic puncture of tissue with subsequent promotion of

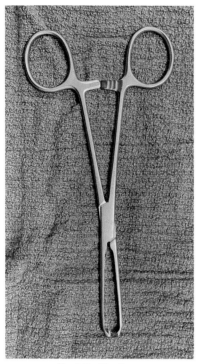

Fig. 2.21 Allis clamp.

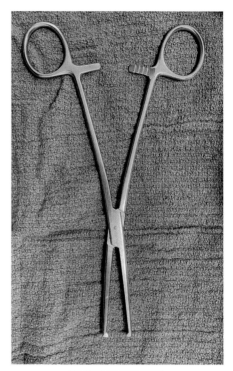

Fig. 2.22 Kocher clamp.

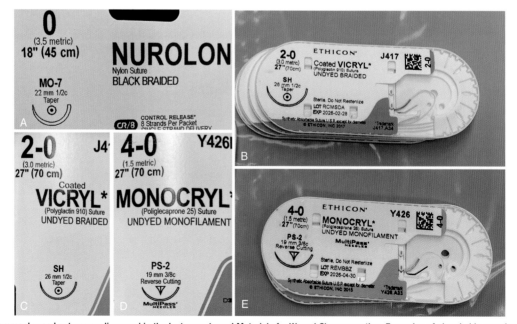

Fig. 2.23 Commonly used sutures as discussed in the Instruments and Materials for Wound Closure section. Examples of absorbable, nonabsorbable, multifilament, and monofilament are shown with their corresponding sizes. (A) Nurolon—a multifilament, nonabsorbable, synthetic suture. (B) Unboxed and (C) boxed Vicryl suture—multifilament, absorbable, synthetic suture. (D) Boxed and (E) unboxed Monocryl suture—monofilament, absorbable, synthetic suture.

scar tissue growth along the closure site. An alternative, or adjunct, to sutures are surgical adhesives.

Adhesives function by allowing in situ polymerization resulting in the adherence of tissue to other tissue, or to nontissue surfaces.[10] In other words they hold two sides of tissue together and support wound healing while the injured tissue heals. Adhesives can be biologically or synthetically derived.

BIOLOGICALLY DERIVED ADHESIVES

The two main biological adhesives are fibrin glue and matrix protein adhesives. Both are derived from human or animal tissues. The benefit of using biological adhesives is that they are biodegradable. A disadvantage is that, relative to synthetic adhesives, there is an increased risk of viral transmission and hypersensitivity reaction.[10] Because of the limited strength of biological adhesives, they are commonly used in addition to sutures rather than alone.

SYNTHETIC ADHESIVES

Cyanoacrylate adhesives (Fig. 2.24) are single-component adhesives that cure in the presence of water or blood

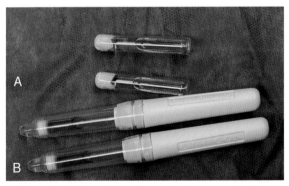

Fig. 2.24 (A) Liquid synthetic surgical adhesive for increased skin adhesion to surgical dressings, Mastisol solution. (B) Synthetic surgical adhesive for wound closure, Dermabond.

at room temperature. They offer tensile strength higher than biological adhesives and similar to that of absorbable sutures.[11]

Failure of cyanoacrylate adhesives is due to the disruption of the skin-glue interface and is more common across joints or in areas with dense hair growth. The wound should be dry prior to application and excess adhesive should be removed with acetone.[12] Some synthetic adhesives have the added benefit of acting as a microbial barrier.[13] Additionally, some adhesives are used for the promotion of a stronger bond between the skin and the overlying surgical dressings covering an incision (Fig. 2.24).

Common synthetic adhesives are listed in Table 2.1.

Closure Instruments

NEEDLE DRIVER

This straight locking clamp is used for holding and manipulating suturing needles. The teeth of the needle driver can be various sizes and are designed to hold the needle in place without any motion of the needle (Fig. 2.25).

ADSON FORCEPS (TOOTHED)

This toothed forceps is used for the precise handling of tissue, especially during closure of the subdermal and dermal layers of the skin (Fig. 2.26).[8]

TOOTHED TISSUE FORCEPS

Similar in function to the Adson forceps, a toothed tissue forceps is slightly larger in size and more commonly used for holding deeper tissue and structures during exposure and closure (Fig. 2.27).

TABLE 2.1 Common Synthetic Adhesives	
Butyl-2-cyanoacrylate adhesives	Indermil (Covidien), Histoacryl and Histoacryl Blue (TissueSeal), and LiquiBand (Advanced Medical Solutions)
Octyl-2-cyanoacrylate adhesives	Dermabond (Ethicon), SurgiSeal (Adhezion Biomedical), LiquiBand Flex (Advanced Medical Solutions), and OctylSeal (Medline Industries)

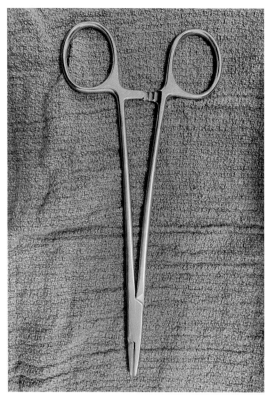

Fig. 2.25 Needle driver.

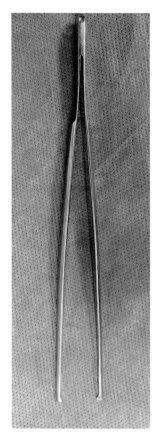

Fig. 2.26 Toothed Adson forceps.

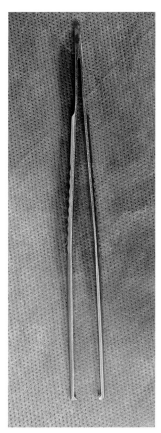

Fig. 2.27 Toothed tissue forceps.

REFERENCES

1. Kreis PG, Fishman S. *Spinal Cord Stimulation: Percutaneous Implantation Techniques*. Oxford, UK: Oxford University Press; 2009.
2. Hay DJ. Electrosurgery. *Surgery (Elsevier)*. 2007;26(2):66-69.
3. Ustatine RP, Pfenninger JL, Stulberg DL, Small R. *Dermatologic and Cosmetic Procedures in Office Practice*. Philadelphia, PA: Elsevier; 2012.
4. Nduka CC, Super PA, Monson JR, Darzi AW. Cause and prevention of electrosurgical injuries in laparoscopy. *J Am Coll Surg*. 1994;179(2):161-170.
5. Aldam P, Pittman H, Haddon R, et al. *History of Anaesthesia Society Proceedings*. vol 45. Wokingham, UK: History of Anaesthesia Society; 2012:1-124.
6. Wu MP, Ou CS, Chen SL, Yen YE, Rowbotham R. Complications and recommended practices for electrosurgery in laparoscopy. *Am J Surg*. 2000;179(1):67-73.
7. Petro C. Basics of Spinal Instruments [Internet]. Basics of Spinal Instruments. Aesculaf Academy; 2014. Available from: https://myhspa.org/images/Lesson_Plans/CIS_Plans/CIS246.pdf. Accessed September 2021.
8. Visenio MR. Commonly Used Surgical Instruments. [Internet]. American College of Surgery; 2018. Available from: https://www.facs.org/media/wgcmalet/common_surgical_instruments_module.pdf. Accessed September 2021.
9. Byrne M, Aly A. The surgical suture. *Aesthet Surg J*. 2019;39(suppl 2):S67-S72.
10. Duarte AP, Coelho JF, Bordado JC, Cidade MT, Gil MH. Surgical adhesives: systematic review of the main types and development forecast. *Prog Polym Sci*. 2012;37:1031-1050.
11. Pan HW, Zhong JX, Jing CX. Comparison of fibrin glue versus suture for conjunctival autografting in pterygium surgery: a meta-analysis. *Ophthalmology*. 2011;118(6):1049-1054.
12. Shapiro AJ, Dinsmore RC, North JH Jr. Tensile strength of wound closure with cyanoacrylate glue. *Am Surg*. 2001;67(11):1113-1115.
13. Bhende S, Rothenburger S, Spangler DJ, Dito M. In vitro assessment of microbial barrier properties of Dermabond topical skin adhesive. *Surg Infect (Larchmt)*. 2002;3(3):251-257.

Chapter 3

Patient Selection for Minimally Invasive Spine Surgery

Jay Darji, Jason Hamamoto, and Behnum Habibi

Introduction

Low back pain is a common health problem suffered by millions of people worldwide and a substantial contributor to disability, affecting individual general well-being and years lived with disability (YLD). In the United States, an estimated 149 million work days are lost every year because of low back pain, with total costs estimated to be $100 to $200 billion per year (of which two-thirds is due to lost wages and lower productivity).[1,2] According to a National Health and Nutrition Examination Survey (NHANES) from 2010, point prevalence for chronic low back pain was 13.1%, with the highest likelihood in the fifth and sixth decades of life.[3] The proportion of people that experience low back pain during their lifetime ranges from 60% to 80%, and a report by Hurwitz et al. estimated that in 2015 roughly 500 million people globally experienced low back pain of at least 3 months duration.[4-7]

There are many risk factors that have an impact on chronic low back pain including age, gender, socioeconomic status, race, general health, occupation, and education level. Women are more likely to have chronic low back pain than men, those who are White are 1.5 times more likely than African Americans or Hispanics to have chronic low back pain, and those with chronic low back pain are less likely to have a college education.[3]

Compared with open spine surgery, minimally invasive spine surgery (MISS) has better cosmetic results from smaller skin incisions (sometimes as small as several millimeters). There is also less blood loss, reduced risk of muscle damage, reduced risk of infection and postoperative pain, faster recovery from surgery with less rehabilitation required, and diminished reliance on pain medications after surgery.[8] In particular, transforaminal interbody lumbar fusion (TLIF) reduces the 2-year societal cost for spine surgeries, causes fewer medical complications, reduces time to return to work, and improves short-term Oswestry Disability Index (ODI) scores.[8]

Patient perception of MISS compared with open surgery also plays an important role in choosing treatment. The most important criteria for patients choosing between open surgery and MISS are long-term outcomes, surgeon's recommendations, and complication risks.[9] When compared with MISS, the majority of patients perceive open surgery to be more painful (83.8%), to have an increased complication risk (78.5%), to have an increased recovery time (89.3%), to have increased costs (68.1%), and to require heavier sedation (62.6%). If required to have spine surgery in the future, the majority of patients prefer a minimally invasive approach (80.0%).[9]

Indications

The indications for MISS are broad and include, but are not limited to:
- degenerative disc disease
- herniated disc
- lumbar spinal stenosis
- spinal deformities such as scoliosis
- spinal infections
- spinal instability including spondylolisthesis
- vertebral compression fractures
- spinal tumors

A more detailed description of indications for MISS follows in the "Patient History" section of this chapter.

Contraindications

As with any medical intervention, risks must be weighed against benefits. MISS can offer select patients with alternatives to undergoing open surgical procedures. There are, however, contraindications for MISS including, but not limited to[10]:

- patients with active infections
- nerve root pathology
- extensive epidural scarring
- abnormal vascular anatomy
- previous retroperitoneal surgery
- severe osteoporosis

Patient History

The indications for minimally invasive spinal fusion (MISF) are broad and include degenerative disease, spondylolisthesis, trauma, spinal deformities, and tumors; therefore candidates may present with a wide range of symptoms.

The patient's history should include questions to assess the quality of the pain and its impact on the patient's daily activities, including nighttime pain that interferes with sleep. Identifying the mechanism of injury is essential if there is an inciting event. However, symptoms may also develop insidiously. The clinician must ask the patient about any current or past treatments, bladder or bowel incontinence, saddle anesthesia, history of malignancy, inflammatory conditions, infections, history of immunosuppression, and drug use. A comprehensive review of systems may reveal red flag signs that suggest underlying infection, inflammatory disease, or malignancy, such as fever, night sweats, or unintentional weight loss.[11]

Patients with disc herniations are generally younger, typically 30 to 50 years old, and have a history of an acute inciting event such as lifting a heavy object, bending, or twisting motions.[12] They may experience localized back pain with associated radicular pain in the arms or legs depending on the location of the herniation (cervical vs. lumbar). There may be weakness, numbness, or paresthesia in specific nerve root distributions due to mechanical and/or chemical irritation of an adjacent nerve root. Patients may also have limited trunk flexion and pain exacerbated by straining, sneezing, and coughing. Seated positioning also worsens pain because of increased pressure applied to the disc.[11] It is also important to inspect the circulatory system, as vascular claudication may mimic neurogenic pathology.

Lumbar spinal stenosis is the most common indication for lumbar spine surgery in patients over 65 years old.[13] Lumbar spinal stenosis classically presents as pain exacerbated by prolonged ambulation, standing upright, and low back extension, owing to the degenerated intervertebral discs, hypertrophy of the facet joints, and thickening of the ligamentum flavum protruding into the spinal canal.[14] The pain is relieved by forward flexion and rest. Neurogenic claudication is an important characteristic of lumbar spinal stenosis. Symptoms are typically bilateral, but usually asymmetric involving the back, buttock, and legs. Pain in addition to numbness and tingling is present in most patients. Symptoms of numbness and tingling typically involve the entire leg and rarely affect an isolated nerve root distribution.[15] Patients may report that walking upstairs is easier than downstairs, as the back is forward flexed with ascending stairs. If patients present with new-onset bowel or bladder dysfunction, bilateral lower extremity weakness, and saddle anesthesia, they may have developed cauda equina syndrome requiring emergent surgical decompression.

Patients with symptomatic spondylolisthesis may present similarly to those affected by spinal stenosis, given that symptoms arise when translation of the vertebral body compresses neural elements from canal narrowing. The clinician should pay special attention to any history of trauma when evaluating for spondylolisthesis, as pars interarticularis defects result from chronic repetitive loading in hyperextension or acute trauma. Low-grade slips and canal stenosis may decompress with forward flexion or sitting, leading to pain relief. As in spinal stenosis, pushing a grocery cart or walking upstairs results in flexion of the spinal column and thereby pain relief.[16] Classically, patients complain of pain that radiates to the buttocks and both lower extremities. If the spondylolisthesis becomes unstable, as evidenced by progression on lateral flexion and extension x-rays, surgery is indicated.

The most common etiology of vertebral compression fractures is osteoporosis, and therefore it is the most common fragility fracture. Vertebral compression fractures demonstrate a bimodal age distribution, as younger patients sustain these injuries from high-energy trauma such as motor vehicle accidents or fall from height. Once the patient has been stabilized, the initial evaluation of spine fractures includes assessment of the neurologic function of the upper and lower extremities, bladder, and bowel. Many high-energy compression fractures have associated abdominal, cerebral, and extremity injuries.

There are many adults who suffer from spinal deformities, such as scoliosis, and live with significant pain and many comorbidities. Open surgical procedures to correct these deformities can be risky, sometimes requiring extensive surgical reconstruction to correct the deformity. Less invasive surgical options can help reduce the risk of complications. Mummaneni et al. previously developed a minimally invasive surgery deformity algorithm (MISDEF) for selection of patients to undergo MISS.[17] These patients were selected based on sagittal parameters, and those with higher degrees of imbalance were not selected. This algorithm was revised to incorporate newer technique options, known as minimally invasive spinal deformity algorithm 2 (MISDEF2).[17] In this updated algorithm, patients are grouped in classes I through IV, compared with previously being grouped in classes I to III. Patients are first grouped according to whether their deformity is fixed or flexible and subsequently on presence or absence of sagittal and coronal deformities.

Physical Examination

When evaluating candidates for MISS, the physical examination should be focused yet broad enough to capture subtle findings related to spinal pathology including pain, postural changes, and gait abnormalities. The curvature of the spine should be assessed to evaluate for loss of lordosis in the cervical and lumbar region indicating degeneration. A scoliosis deformity may be observed, or the patient may have a high steppage gait to avoid toe drag owing to foot drop. Abnormal limb advancement may indicate pain in the back or extremities from nerve root compression.

The range of motion (ROM) examination of the neck and back is important to assess because loss of ROM and pain elicited in specific planes can help localize the lesion. Normal cervical spine ROM is 0 to 45 degrees of flexion and extension, 0 to 70 degrees of rotation, and 0 to 40 degrees of lateral bending.[18]

Lumbar spine ROM is assessed with the patient in a standing position and should be observed with the practitioner at the back or side of the patient. The practitioner may stabilize the patient by placing their hands on the pelvis to ensure that motion only occurs at the spine. Motion occurs in three planes and includes four directions, as follows: forward flexion—52 degrees ±9; extension—19 degrees ±9; lateral flexion/side bending—31 degrees ±6; rotation—32 degrees ±9.[19]

Palpation of the spine helps to identify focal tenderness from muscles, tendons, ligaments, and joints. The examiner should begin at the cervical region including the shoulders then work down to the lumbosacral region including the sacroiliac joints. Severe point tenderness may suggest the presence of a fracture or underlying infection such as an epidural abscess.[20] It is important to note a palpable step-off deformity, which may be present in the setting of an acute trauma or severe spondylolisthesis.

Muscle strength testing is performed to evaluate for muscle weakness from a neurologic deficit, poor endurance, or muscle imbalance. Strength can be evaluated in multiple ways including manual muscle testing or functional strength testing. The most accepted method of evaluating muscle strength is the Medical Research Council Manual Muscle Testing scale that tests key muscles of the upper and lower extremities against the examiner's resistance.[21] Strength is graded on a scale of 0 to 5, and commonly tested key muscles and the corresponding spinal nerve roots include:

- Upper extremity
  - Shoulder abductors
  - Elbow flexors (biceps, brachialis)—C5
  - Wrist extensors (extensor carpi radialis longus and brevis)—C6
  - Elbow extensors (triceps)—C7
  - Finger flexors (flexor digitorum profundus)—C8
  - Hand intrinsics (abductor digiti minimi)—T1
- Lower extremity
  - Hip flexors (iliopsoas)—L2
  - Knee extensors (quadriceps)—L3
  - Ankle dorsiflexors (tibialis anterior)—L4
  - Great toe extensor (extensor hallucis longus)—L5

- Ankle plantar flexors (gastrocnemius, soleus)—S1

Functional muscle testing provides a more dynamic assessment of strength and allows muscles to work synergistically as intended physiologically. Proximal lower extremity strength can be tested by having a patient rise from a seated chair position without the use of their arms or performing a double leg squat. The single leg squat also tests muscular asymmetry in addition to strength as medial knee deviation or pelvic tilt indicates proximal muscle issues. Heel walking and toe walking assesses distal muscle strength including ankle dorsiflexors and plantar flexors.

Sensory testing of the upper and lower extremities is necessary to evaluate spinal nerve roots and peripheral nerves to further localize the lesion. For practical purposes, testing sensation to light touch using the examiner's digits or a cotton wisp is used as a clinical screening tool and lesions can be localized to different human dermatomes as represented in Fig. 3.1. If an impairment is identified, then further tests may be performed. Proprioception is tested by moving the distal phalanges of the hands and feet up and down with the patient's eyes closed to assess if they can sense the position of the joint. If the patient cannot, then the examiner may test a more proximal joint.

Muscle stretch reflexes are important to evaluate and provide information on the possible presence of upper or lower motor neuron disease. There are five commonly tested reflexes that include the biceps (C5–C6), brachioradialis (C6), triceps (C7–C8), patellar (L2–L4), and Achilles (S1–S2). The National Institute of Neurological Disorders and Stroke (NINDS) proposed a grading scale from 0 to 4 to classify the reflex response.[22] Special attention should be paid to any asymmetry of the reflex response as this is suggestive of underlying pathology. Additionally, upper motor neuron signs should be evaluated to assess for myelopathy, which include the Hoffman reflex, Babinski reflex, ankle clonus, and increased muscular tone.

SPECIAL TESTS
Cervical Spine

Spurling test is performed with the patient sitting upright and extending their neck to 30 degrees and looking to one side while the examiner applies an axial load on their head to compress the neural foramen on the ipsilateral side of head rotation. A positive test is reproduced pain/numbness into the arm in a radicular distribution suggesting cervical radiculopathy. Spurling test is very specific (93%) with low sensitivity; therefore it is helpful in confirming the diagnosis of cervical radiculopathy.[23]

Cervical distraction is performed with the patient sitting upright or lying supine and the examiner placing their hands around the mastoid processes to pull and apply a distraction force to widen the neural foramina bilaterally. A positive test is when the patient's radicular pain is alleviated with traction, suggesting cervical radiculopathy.[24]

Lhermitte sign describes a transient electric shock sensation down the upper extremities and spine elicited with neck flexion, which is classically associated with multiple sclerosis but may also be present in myelopathy and radiculopathy.

Bakody sign, also known as the shoulder abduction test, is noted when the patient performs active shoulder abduction of their symptomatic arm and places it on their head, which releases traction on the cervical nerve roots, particularly C4–C6, leading to pain relief. This is suggestive of cervical radiculopathy.[24]

Lumbar Spine

Kemp test, also known as the lumbar facet grind test, is performed with the patient standing and arms crossed at the chest. The examiner then stands behind the patient and places one hand on the pelvis and another on the shoulder and extends the patient's lumbar spine 30 degrees and laterally rotates to both sides while applying a downward axial force. Axial pain at maximal extension and rotation indicates a positive test suggesting lumbar facet arthropathy ipsilateral to the side of rotation.

The straight leg raise test is performed with the patient lying supine while the examiner raises one leg slowly up to 70 degrees keeping the contralateral leg and pelvis down on the table. A positive test is the reproduction of pain or numbness radiating into the leg at 30 to 70 degrees of elevation, indicating lumbosacral nerve root irritation.

The seated slump test is performed with the patient seated at the edge of the exam table with their trunk slumped into flexion. The examiner applies

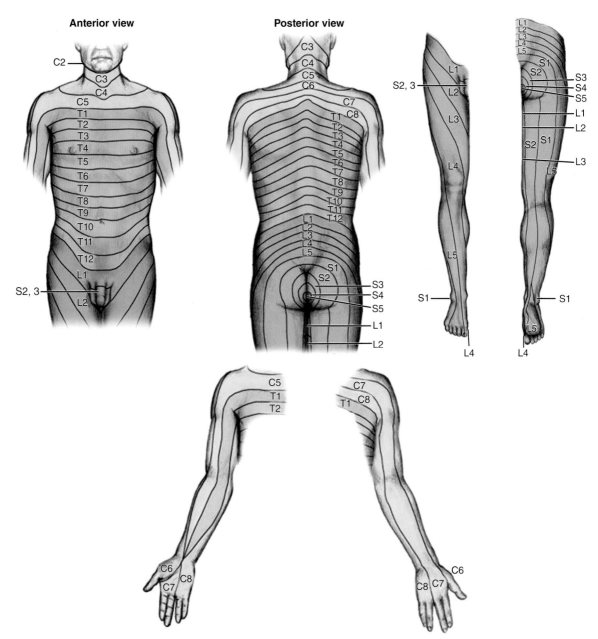

Fig. 3.1 Dermatome map. (From Tubbs RS, Rizk E, Shoja M, Loukas M, Barbaro N, Spinner RJ. *Nerves and Nerve Injuries.* Vol. 1. History, Embryology, Anatomy, Imaging, and Diagnostics. Academic Press; 2015: 477-478).

gentle pressure on their head and raises the hip into 90 degrees of flexion and knee into full extension by grasping the ankle. A positive test is reproduction of pain in the low back and lower extremities indicating radiculopathy or sciatic nerve irritation.[18] The pain should resolve when neck and trunk flexion is released.

The femoral nerve stretch test is performed with the patient lying prone with the knee flexed. The examiner extends the patient's hip while maintaining knee flexion. A positive test is pain or numbness in the anterior thigh or back, which indicates femoral nerve irritation or lumbar radiculopathy.[18]

Previously Failed Treatments

Before undergoing MISS, patients should try a multitude of conservative measures. Treatment options include physical therapy to strengthen the surrounding musculature to stabilize the spinal column, as well as improve flexibility to reduce stress on joints. Oral medications may be used to manage painful symptoms. Bracing is another conservative option to provide support to the spine and offload the facet joints and intervertebral discs. Epidural steroid injections are another treatment option to help temporize a patient's symptoms, and multiple approaches may be used, including transforaminal and interlaminar.

Conclusion

MISS offers patients an alternative to open surgery and, in many cases, a last resort after failed previous treatment methods. There are numerous indications for MISS including spinal stenosis, degenerative disc disease, disc herniations, spondylolisthesis, and spinal deformities; however, patients must have a well-documented physical exam along with an understanding of the risks and benefits of MISS. As with any intervention, there are contraindications to MISS that include, but are not limited to, infections, nerve root pathology, abnormal vascular anatomy, and severe osteoporosis. When compared with open surgery, MISS is perceived by patients to provide benefits such as lower complication risk, shorter recovery time, lower cost, and less pain. Future studies should continue to evaluate these perceived benefits.

REFERENCES

1. Katz JN. Lumbar disc disorders and low-back pain: socioeconomic factors and consequences. *J Bone Joint Surg Am.* 2006;88(suppl 2):21-24.
2. Rubin DI. Epidemiology and risk factors for spine pain. *Neurol Clin.* 2007;25(2):353-371.
3. Shmagel A, Foley R, Ibrahim H. Epidemiology of chronic low back pain in US adults: data from the 2009-2010 National Health and Nutrition Examination Survey. *Arthritis Care Res (Hoboken).* 2016;68(11):1688-1694.
4. Hurwitz EL, Randhawa K, Yu H, Cote P, Haldeman S. The Global Spine Care Initiative: a summary of the global burden of low back and neck pain studies. *Eur Spine J.* 2018;27(suppl 6):796-801.
5. Hoy D, March L, Brooks P, et al. The global burden of low back pain: estimates from the Global Burden of Disease 2010 study. *Ann Rheum Dis.* 2014;73(6):968-974.
6. Driscoll T, Jacklyn G, Orchard J, et al. The global burden of occupationally related low back pain: estimates from the Global Burden of Disease 2010 study. *Ann Rheum Dis.* 2014;73(6):975-981.
7. Reveille JD, Weisman MH. The epidemiology of back pain, axial spondyloarthritis and HLA-B27 in the United States. *Am J Med Sci.* 2013;345(6):431-436.
8. McClelland S III, Goldstein JA. Minimally invasive versus open spine surgery: what does the best evidence tell us? *J Neurosci Rural Pract.* 2017;8(2):194-198.
9. Narain AS, Hijji FY, Duhancioglu G, et al. Patient perceptions of minimally invasive versus open spine surgery. *Clin Spine Surg.* 2018;31(3):E184-E192.
10. Allain J, Dufour T. Anterior lumbar fusion techniques: ALIF, OLIF, DLIF, LLIF, IXLIF. *Orthop Traumatol Surg Res.* 2020;106(suppl 1):S149-S157.
11. Amin RM, Andrade NS, Neuman BJ. Lumbar disc herniation. *Curr Rev Musculoskelet Med.* 2017;10(4):507-516.
12. Fjeld OR, Grøvle L, Helgeland J, et al. Complications, reoperations, readmissions, and length of hospital stay in 34 639 surgical cases of lumbar disc herniation. *Bone Joint J.* 2019;101-B(4):470-477.
13. Zaina F, Tomkins-Lane C, Carragee E, Negrini S. Surgical versus nonsurgical treatment for lumbar spinal stenosis. *Spine (Phila Pa 1976).* 2016;41(14):E857-E868.
14. Alvarez JA, Hardy RH Jr. Lumbar spine stenosis: a common cause of back and leg pain. *Am Fam Physician.* 1998;57(8):1825-1834, 1839-1840.
15. Hall S, Bartleson JD, Onofrio BM, Baker HL Jr, Okazaki H, O'Duffy JD. Lumbar spinal stenosis. Clinical features, diagnostic procedures, and results of surgical treatment in 68 patients. *Ann Intern Med.* 1985;103(2):271-275.
16. Syrmou E, Tsitsopoulos PP, Marinopoulos D, Tsonidis C, Anagnostopoulos I, Tsitsopoulos PD. Spondylolysis: a review and reappraisal. *Hippokratia.* 2010;14(1):17-21.
17. Mummaneni PV, Park P, Shaffrey CI, et al. The MISDEF2 algorithm: an updated algorithm for patient selection in minimally invasive deformity surgery. *J Neurosurg Spine.* 2019;32(2):221-228.
18. Miller A, Heckert KD, Davis BA. *The 3-Minute Musculoskeletal and Peripheral Nerve Exam.* 1st ed. Demos Medical; 2009.
19. Ng JK, Kippers V, Richardson C, Parnianpour M. Range of motion and lordosis of the lumbar spine. *Spine.* 2001;26(1):53-60.
20. Bratton RL. Assessment and management of acute low back pain. *Am Fam Physician.* 1999;60(8):2299-2308.
21. Williams M. Manual muscle testing, development and current use. *Phys Ther Rev.* 1956;36(12):797-805.
22. Hallett M. NINDS myotatic reflex scale. *Neurology.* 1993;43(12):2723.
23. Tong HC, Haig AJ, Yamakawa K. The Spurling test and cervical radiculopathy. *Spine (Phila Pa 1976).* 2002;27(2):156-159.
24. Malanga GA, Landes P, Nadler SF. Provocative tests in cervical spine examination: historical basis and scientific analyses. *Pain Physician.* 2003;6(2):199-205.

Chapter 4

Perioperative Management and Best Practices

Ryan Steven D'Souza and Alaa Abd-Elsayed

Introduction

As evidence grows for the benefits of percutaneous fusion procedures in the treatment of mechanical low back pain, it is important for the proceduralist to pursue appropriate workup and assess for proper patient selection. Poor patient selection and inadequate preoperative workup may lead to suboptimal long-term results and may increase risk for perioperative complications. Although there are no current established guidelines for perioperative workup in patients who are candidates for percutaneous fusion procedures, we recommend adherence to guidelines commonly used for other neuraxial interventions such as spinal cord stimulator placement. This is justified, as a conservative standard is adhered to as evidence and guidelines continue to evolve for percutaneous fusion procedures. In addition, many percutaneous fusion procedures are performed close to the neuraxial space and thus carry similar risks to other neuraxial interventions. In this chapter, we provide a summary of recommendations that should be undertaken in the preoperative, intraoperative, and postoperative period in patients pursuing percutaneous fusion procedures.

Preoperative Care

ASSESSMENT OF CLINICAL INDICATION

First, the clinician should confirm that the patient has an appropriate clinical indication to benefit from a percutaneous fusion procedure. For example, if the patient is offered a percutaneous facet joint fusion procedure, the patient should have one of the following diagnoses: facet joint dysfunction and pain, spinal instability from prior spine surgeries, microinstability

of certain spinal segments, or requirement for adjunctive therapy or bridging therapy to an interbody fusion surgery. Clinical indications for other percutaneous fusion procedures are presented elsewhere within this atlas. A thorough assessment of contraindications that would preclude the proceduralist from offering this therapy to the patient should be reviewed, including coagulopathy, current infection, malignancy, and other contraindications.

Another essential component in the preoperative period is for the patient to have an "education" visit, where all questions relevant to the surgery are addressed. In many centers with specialized pain practices, this is often conducted by a nurse or an advanced nurse practitioner. This visit presents an opportunity for the patient to visualize the type of device that would be implanted, discuss alternative or adjunctive treatment, potentially meet with the device company representative, and address any pending questions before the surgery.

PSYCHIATRIC SCREENING VISIT

The biopsychosocial approach to chronic pain management involves a complex interaction between biological, psychological, social, and medicolegal factors. It is well-known that chronic pain and mood disorders often cooccur, as highlighted by studies citing that up to 85% of chronic pain patients are impacted by severe depression.[1,2] Furthermore, chronic pain patients who suffer from uncontrolled mood disorder exhibit a poorer prognosis than patients who have chronic pain only.[3] Thus it is not uncommon for the proceduralist to obtain a presurgical psychological assessment of patients before offering them advanced interventional options. Presurgical psychosocial health is a major predictor of pain relief, quality of life, and satisfaction after spinal cord stimulator placement.[4,5] Thus although a patient may appear to be an ideal candidate for a surgery based on their clinical indication, poorly controlled psychological comorbidities may make them suboptimal candidates. Furthermore, even other psychosocial factors, such as history of drug abuse, alcoholism, personality issues, marital discord, job dissatisfaction, pending litigation, and prior abuse or abandonment, may play a role in a patient's postsurgical efficacy. Thus a preoperative general psychosocial assessment should include a survey of pain symptoms, demographic data, prior surgeries, employment status, level of education, history of workers' compensation or other injury litigation, disability payment status, and personality traits.

IMAGING STUDIES

Preoperative advanced imaging of the surgical area of interest, utilizing either computed tomography (CT) or magnetic resonance imaging (MRI), is recommended for presurgical planning, to rule out any contraindications or anatomic abnormalities that would preclude the proceduralist from offering percutaneous fusion, and to minimize risk of complications. This imaging should be recent to within 1 to 2 years of the planned procedure. Spine surgeons typically utilize preoperative multiplanar advanced imaging to inform medical decisions and surgical plans before spine fusion surgery that involves pedicle screw instrumentation.[6] Similarly, in the neuromodulation space, obtaining preoperative thoracic MRI for thoracic lead placement is the standard of care and has been recommended by consensus committees.[7] Thus the authors recommend obtaining either an MRI or CT scan before performing percutaneous fusion procedures.

In addition, osteoporosis has often been considered as a contraindication to spine surgeries that involve instrumentation.[8] Studies have demonstrated that patients with substantially lower bone mineral density are at high risk for developing graft subsidence, failure of spinal fusion and implant fixation, and vertebral compression fractures surrounding fusion sites.[9,10] Presurgical optimization with bisphosphonates may lead to improved outcomes including increased solid intervertebral fusion, decreased vertebral compression fractures, decreased pedicle screw loosening, and decreased case subsidence.[10] Obtaining a presurgical bone density scan, such as a dual-energy x-ray absorptiometry (DEXA) scan, may help inform this decision.

ANTICOAGULATION

Many percutaneous fusion procedures are in proximity to the neuraxial space and are thus considered as high-to-intermediate risk procedures. Anticoagulation should be held with approval of the prescribing physician for an adequate length of time specific for the anticoagulant medication, before the procedure. Commonly, proceduralists follow anticoagulation practice guidelines as stated by the American Society of Regional Anesthesia and Pain Medicine Consensus committee.[11,12] Proceduralists may also choose to follow consensus guidelines that are in place for spinal cord stimulator placement.[13] Generally, nonsteroidal antiinflammatory drugs, other antiplatelet agents, and anticoagulants should be discontinued for at least five half-lives. Furthermore, depending on the patient's bleeding risk, medical comorbidities (e.g., renal or hepatic dysfunction), and the type of anticoagulant, proceduralists may also consider obtaining diagnostic workup that includes hemoglobin, platelet count, prothrombin time, international normalized ratio, and partial thromboplastin time.

In settings where a patient is at high risk for a thromboembolic event, a shared assessment and risk stratification approach between the proceduralist and the provider who prescribes anticoagulation is warranted. High-risk patients who require bridging of anticoagulation therapy may be bridged with low-molecular-weight heparin or heparin. Proceduralists may consider consulting with a vascular medicine service if a thrombophilia specialty service is available to assist in anticoagulation management perioperatively.

OTHER PREOPERATIVE RECOMMENDATIONS

Optimal glucose control is recommended, and most guidelines advise a hemoglobin A1c level below 8% to 9%.[14] Tobacco cessation is also recommended, as continued use may impair surgical healing. Patients who are carriers of methicillin-sensitive *Staphylococcus aureus* (MSSA) and methicillin-resistant *S. aureus* (MRSA) should receive mupirocin nasal ointment and chlorhexidine baths for decolonization.[15]

Intraoperative Care

INFECTION PREVENTION

Strict sterile precautions are recommended intraoperatively. This entails performing a surgical scrub for 2 to 5 minutes with an antiseptic, wearing a surgical mask, wearing a sterile gown and double gloves, using chlorhexidine gluconate for preoperative skin preparation, placing an iodophor-impregnated drape, removing hair near surgical site with electric clippers, and using laminar flow and high-efficiency particulate air (HEPA) filters in the operating room.[15] Administration of prophylactic antibiotics within 1 hour of surgical incision is recommended. Finally, application of a biooclusive dressing after the surgery that remains in place for 24 to 48 hours is recommended.

Postoperative Care

INFECTION PREVENTION

The key tenet of infection prevention is adherence to the prescribed postoperative antibiotic regimen. Although antibiotic prescription practices vary considerably among providers, recent guidelines for spinal cord stimulator procedures recommend postoperative antibiotics for 24 hours. Given the proximity to the neuraxial space of fusion procedures, the authors also recommend at least 24 hours of postoperative antibiotic therapy.

Furthermore, patients should not shower or remove wound dressings for 48 hours. After that, dressing changes can occur daily. Dressings may be removed before showering, and then incisions should be patted dry and allowed to air dry after showering, with subsequent replacement of dressing. Patients should refrain from completely submerging under water, such as in baths, hot tubs, or swimming pools, for at least 2 weeks. Finally, the patient should monitor for any signs or symptoms that would be concerning for infection such as worsening incisional pain, erythema over the incision, swelling, fever, or pus-like discharge from the incision.

POSTOPERATIVE RESUMPTION OF ANTICOAGULATION

When resuming antiplatelet and anticoagulation agents after percutaneous fusion, proceduralists should adhere to practice guidelines from the American Society of Regional Anesthesia and Pain Medicine Consensus committee.[11,12] Aspirin may be resumed after 24 hours, and clopidogrel may be resumed after 12 to 24 hours. Warfarin may be restarted 6 hours postoperatively. All novel oral anticoagulants (NOACs) should be restarted 24 hours postoperatively. Exceptions to standard care should be individualized and should be made through expert consultation with the vascular medicine service.

INCISIONAL PAIN CONTROL

Patients should employ a multimodal analgesia protocol to assist with incisional pain. The proceduralist may infiltrate the surgical area with local anesthetic. Barring any contraindications, patients may take acetaminophen and nonsteroidal antiinflammatory agents. Ice application over the incisional area may decrease inflammation and pain. Finally, the proceduralist may prescribe a short, 3- to 5-day course of short-acting opioid medication.

ACTIVITY RESTRICTIONS

Activity restrictions may vary institutionally, but certain recommendations are consistent. During the first 2 weeks after fusion, patients should refrain from intense physical activity that could impact the implanted hardware such as weight lifting, biking, running, sexual activity, lifting over 5 pounds, and twisting or bending over 30 degrees. The limited movement prevents migration of the implant and allows the incision to appropriately form scar tissue. During weeks 2 through 6, patients may lift up to 10 pounds in weight, but should continue to refrain from bending and twisting the spine. During weeks 6 to 12, most normal daily activities can be resumed although it is still recommended to refrain from high-impact activities such as horseback riding or riding in all-terrain vehicles.

FOLLOW-UP VISITS

Follow-up visits are crucial to address any adverse effects and to monitor treatment efficacy from the surgical intervention. Traditionally, patients would follow up with the proceduralist at postoperative weeks 10 to 14 for inspection of incisions and removal of any superficial closure materials (e.g., staples). Thereafter routine follow-up is at the discretion of the proceduralist, but may occur at 3 months, 6 months, and 1 year postsurgery to monitor for efficacy of treatment.

REFERENCES

1. Buono FD, Savage SR, Cerrito B, et al. Chronic pain, mood disorders and substance use: outcomes of interdisciplinary care in a residential psychiatric hospital. *J Pain Res.* 2020;13: 1515-1523.
2. Williams LS, Jones WJ, Shen J, Robinson RL, Weinberger M, Kroenke K. Prevalence and impact of depression and pain in neurology outpatients. *J Neurol Neurosurg Psychiatry.* 2003; 74(11):1587-1589.
3. Sheng J, Liu S, Wang Y, Cui R, Zhang X. The link between depression and chronic pain: neural mechanisms in the brain. *Neural Plast.* 2017;2017:9724371.
4. Blackburn DR, Romers CC, Copeland LA, et al. Presurgical psychological assessments as correlates of effectiveness of spinal cord stimulation for chronic pain reduction. *Neuromodulation.* 2016;19(4):422-428.
5. Fama CA, Chen N, Prusik J, et al. The use of preoperative psychological evaluations to predict spinal cord stimulation success: our experience and a review of the literature. *Neuromodulation.* 2016;19(4):429-436.
6. Kepler CK, Pavlov H, Kim HJ, Green DW, Rawlins BA. Preoperative templating before spinal fusion using a fluoroscopic multiplanar imaging system is as accurate as CT scan and uses substantially less radiation. *J Pediatr Orthop.* 2012;32(8):e67-e71.
7. Stone LE, Falowski SM. Pre-operative imaging for spinal cord stimulation: a case report of a spinal cord tumor identified by screening magnetic resonance imaging of the thoracic spine. *Neuromodulation.* 2019;22(3):355-357.
8. Tomé-Bermejo F, Piñera AR, Alvarez-Galovich L. Osteoporosis and the management of spinal degenerative disease (I). *Arch Bone Jt Surg.* 2017;5(5):272-282.
9. Tempel ZJ, Gandhoke GS, Okonkwo DO, Kanter AS. Impaired bone mineral density as a predictor of graft subsidence following minimally invasive transpsoas lateral lumbar interbody fusion. *Eur Spine J.* 2015;24(suppl 3):414-419.
10. Liu WB, Zhao WT, Shen P, Zhang FJ. The effects of bisphosphonates on osteoporotic patients after lumbar fusion: a meta-analysis. *Drug Des Devel Ther.* 2018;12:2233-2240.
11. Horlocker TT, Wedel DJ, Rowlingson JC, et al. Regional anesthesia in the patient receiving antithrombotic or thrombolytic therapy: American Society of Regional Anesthesia and Pain Medicine evidence-based guidelines (third edition). *Reg Anesth Pain Med.* 2010;35(1):64-101.
12. Narouze S, Benzon HT, Provenzano D, et al. Interventional spine and pain procedures in patients on antiplatelet and anticoagulant medications (second edition): guidelines from the American Society of Regional Anesthesia and Pain Medicine, the European Society of Regional Anaesthesia and Pain Therapy, the American Academy of Pain Medicine, the International Neuromodulation Society, the North American Neuromodulation Society, and the World Institute of Pain. *Reg Anesth Pain Med.* 2018;43(3):225-262.
13. Deer TR, Narouze S, Provenzano DA, et al. The Neurostimulation Appropriateness Consensus Committee (NACC): recommendations on bleeding and coagulation management in neurostimulation devices. *Neuromodulation.* 2017;20(1):51-62.
14. Akiboye F, Rayman G. Management of hyperglycemia and diabetes in orthopedic surgery. *Curr Diab Rep.* 2017;17(2):13.
15. Deer TR, Provenzano DA, Hanes M, et al. The Neurostimulation Appropriateness Consensus Committee (NACC) recommendations for infection prevention and management. *Neuromodulation.* 2017;20(1):31-50.

Chapter 5

Minimally Invasive Posterior Lumbar Fusion—A Novel Approach to Facet Fusion

Michael Gyorfi, Omar Viswanath, and Alaa Abd-Elsayed

Introduction

Facet fusion, or posterior lumbar fusion (PLF), is one of the oldest treatments for chronic back pain. From the earliest types of fusion in the late 1800s through modern-day technologies such as facet screws, bone grafts, and interbody devices, there have been significant advancements in technique and instrumentation.[1]

History

First, in 1911, Albee created a primitive version of a PLF. In 1944 King described a procedure that included a crude posterior fusion with facet screws that crossed the facet joint.[2] Then in 1953 Watkins and Campbell pioneered the contemporary style of PLF, which comprised fusing the facet joints, pars interarticularis, and bases of the transverse processes.[3] It was not until the 1970s that a specialized treatment for facet joint discomfort was developed, and facet pain had been mostly ignored until then.[4] Magerl was the first to use translaminar facet screws (TLFSs) in 1983.[2]

Facet screw fixation has become a standard treatment, but the methods and practice of combining it with fusion techniques have progressed. Until recently, doctors would dissect all the tissue from the posterior components of the vertebrae implicated in the fusion (including fascia, ligaments, and muscle). This included both vertebrae's transverse processes, the lateral facet joints, and possibly the lateral lamina. Decortication (removal of the bony cortex) is conducted after this extensive dissection is completed, by grinding the outer covering (the cortex) off these bones to prepare the area for fusion. The exposed bone is required to provide blood, mesenchymal stem cells, and growth factors to the bone graft for fusion to occur. All three of these components are required for healing, as they offer osteoinduction, osteoconduction, and osteogenesis.[5] Today, a new approach allows for the same bone decortication as before, but without the need for substantial tissue dissection. With advancements in medical technology, physicians can now execute this surgery in a less invasive manner, potentially reducing blood loss, scarring, and recovery time.

Facet-Mediated Low Back Pain

Facet-mediated low back pain is thought to account for 25% to 40% of all low back pain.[6] With neighboring-level pathology from earlier fusions or spinal operations, this number rises even more. Kyphoplasty and spinal augmentation operations are two procedures that may aggravate facet discomfort. Disc degeneration, spondylolisthesis, inflammatory arthritis, instability, and traumatic injuries are all diseases that can cause facet-mediated low back pain.[7] On a magnetic resonance imaging (MRI) or computed tomography (CT) scan, these findings can be seen as a facet cyst or facet arthritic changes. Prior surgery at the same level is responsible for a smaller subset of facet-mediated pain. Interspinous spacers and other spinal implants aid in resisting motion in flexion and extension, but they do not help with lateral bending or axial rotation. Facet joints may stay flexible, and facet pain may last for a long time. To diagnose this as a pain modulator, an MRI or diagnostic blocks of the facet joints are frequently required (Fig. 5.1). After surgery, the joint can become weakened, leading to arthritic changes or abnormal mobility, resulting in facet-mediated discomfort.

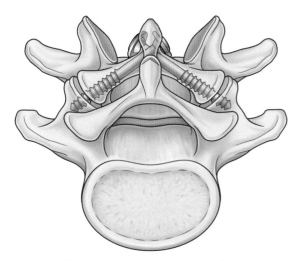

Fig. 5.1 Translaminar facet screw fixation.

Facet-mediated low back pain is a common cause of disability. Common causes of facet-mediated low back pain include:

- Repetitively lifting heavy objects
- Sudden flexion-extension injury from a motor vehicle accident
- Excessive strain on the muscles from prolonged sitting or incorrect positioning
- Prolonged use of high-heeled shoes
- Poor posture
- Obesity
- Sports injuries
- Prior surgical intervention

Understanding the anatomy of the lumbar spine is necessary to comprehend the natural history of facet-mediated back pain. Although most adults have five lumbar vertebrae, it is estimated that about 5% of adults have a sixth lumbar vertebrae.[8] In a healthy person, this is known as a transitional vertebra and should not pose any problems. The lumbar disc is located between the lumbar vertebrae. Patients who have had one of the aforementioned events may develop low back pain over time. This is most commonly, but not always, the outcome of anterior column disc degeneration and loss of integrity. Facet joints may become a source of pain if the disc is unable to maintain the tension across the lower back.[9] The facet joints located in the lumbar spine (Fig. 5.2) are most susceptible to facet damage, as the lumbar spine bears the most weight and endures the greatest amount of stress/strain. Years of tension and exertion can wear down the intervertebral discs and facet joints. Water is the biggest constituent of an intervertebral disc, and age-related degenerative changes impact disc hydration, resulting in disc height loss and changes in facet joint alignment. Facet joint discomfort can result from this degeneration and misalignment. Facet joint syndrome frequently occurs in the presence of other spinal degenerative illnesses, such as degenerative disc disease, spondylolisthesis, and spondylosis (spinal osteoarthritis), and is a prevalent cause of low back discomfort. The lower back, as well as the buttocks and/or thighs, may be painful.[7] Stiffness and difficulties standing up straight or sleeping on a flat surface can be caused by inflammation of these joints. Leaning forward generally relieves problems, whereas extension often aggravates them.

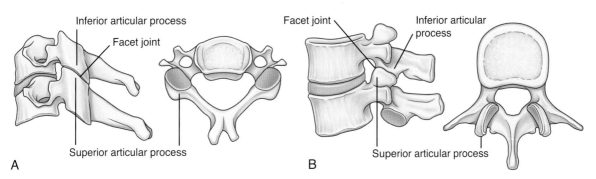

Fig. 5.2 (A) Cervical and (B) lumbar facet joint anatomy.

Anatomy and Biomechanics of the Facet Joints

The zygapophyseal joints, commonly known as facet joints, are biomechanically complicated joints in the spine. The ranges of motion in flexion, extension, lateral bending, and axial rotation are limited by these joints.[10] They form a motion segment in conjunction with the spinal disc, and the disc and superior/inferior facet joints on the right and left sides make up each motion segment. The facet joint is a synovial joint that secretes synovial fluid to keep it lubricated. Capsular ligaments surround the joints and serve to support the joint capsule. Owing to the strong innervation of medial branch fibers, high stretch values are the likely cause of discomfort when instability occurs.[10] Because of the abnormal gliding of the joints, arthritic joints are also a source of discomfort. In the neuroforamen, spinal nerves exit anterior to the facet joint. Nerves can become squeezed, inducing peripheral neurologic symptoms when osteoarthritis or disc height decrease occurs.

Modern Facet Procedures

The facet joints are operated on to relieve discomfort by stabilizing the mobility segment. TLFS fixation, transfacet screw fixation, and intrafacet bone allograft fusion are the most prevalent procedures used today.[11] Depending on the physician's preference, the three techniques can be performed bilaterally in an open or minimally invasive manner. The key difference between these methods is the trajectory through which the implant is inserted (Fig. 5.3). When it comes to implant safety and efficacy, the trajectory is crucial. The screw must pass across the facet joint and have purchase via the superior articular process and inferior articular process of a facet joint when conducting translaminar facet fixation or transfacet fixation. The screw exerts a compressive stress on the joint, stabilizing it. The implant is inserted into the facet joint during an intrafacet fusion, and it usually contains characteristics that give it purchase within the joint. This approach is popular because it eliminates the need for the implant to pass through any sensitive neurologic structures. The screw must be positioned extremely precisely in a translaminar approach so that the threads do not breach the lamina cortex and enter the vertebral foramen. Another advantage of the intrafacet technique is that it allows for fixing without the use of metallic hardware. The cortex of the articular surfaces of the facet joint is removed in most intrafacet methods, and a cortical bone allograft is implanted. To generate another point of possible fusion across the joint, a bone graft is often placed on top of the implant.

Indications

The major goal of posterior facet arthrodesis treatments is to fuse the identified pain generators, to relieve symptoms and allow the patient to resume

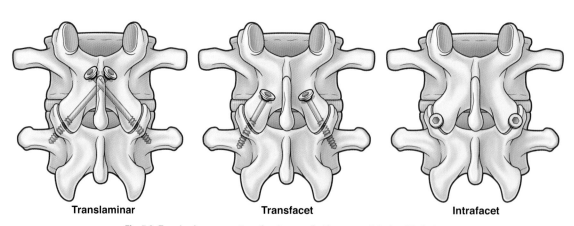

Fig. 5.3 Translaminar versus transfacet screw fixation versus intrafacet trajectory.

Translaminar   Transfacet   Intrafacet

normal activities. Patients who are indicated for this procedure have undergone a workup that has determined that a pain generator is located at the facet joint or joints (Fig. 5.4). Fusion is usually done bilaterally in any circumstance, as it stabilizes and avoids global motions. Before deciding on facet arthrodesis, doctors should make sure the patient has tried conservative treatments, including physical therapy and antiinflammatory medication. It is critical to concentrate on core stabilization and body mass index (BMI) optimization in physical therapy. Patients who do not respond to this treatment plan are frequently given diagnostic and therapeutic facet blocks. To diagnose and treat persistent facet pain, well-established techniques such as facet joint blocks, medial branch blocks, and rhizotomies are employed.[7] Gender, age, and weight all have an impact on the likelihood that the patient's low back discomfort is caused by facet joint pain. Facet joint disease, which results from the accumulative deterioration of the joint, is more common as people get older. If a patient arrives with low back

discomfort, a higher BMI is linked to a higher risk that the discomfort is caused by facet joint pain. The greater weight distributions on the facet joints are the cause of this. Patients who have had past lumbosacral spine procedures are more likely to develop facet joint pain at adjacent levels. These joints are subjected to increased stress and load, which may hasten articular surface deterioration. The disc and facet joints nearby act as shock absorbers and provide a wide range of motion.

Contraindications

- Morbid obesity
- Pregnancy
- Distorted anatomy
- Medical or surgical conditions that may preclude the potential benefit of the procedure
- Rapid joint disease, bone absorption, osteopenia, osteomalacia, and osteoporosis are relative contraindications
- Tumors
- High grade instability
- Grade 2 or higher spondylolisthesis
- Systemic or localized infection
- Inability to lay prone
- Allergy to drugs used in the procedure

Patient Selection

The initial success of almost all operative outcomes is dependent on proper patient selection. The clinician has appropriately diagnosed the etiology of the pain as facet mediated once the abovementioned criteria have been applied and/or exhausted. Although the cause of pain is frequently complicated, facet-mediated low back pain is a curable condition. The following contraindications should be monitored when selecting patients who may not achieve the expected results. Patients with a spondylitic spondylolisthesis or a movable listhesis on flexion or extension views are not recommended. Those who have active infections should also be avoided. Rheumatoid arthritis is not a contraindication. Patients are also encouraged to keep their blood glucose levels in check. Infection is more likely in people who have a hemoglobin A1c of 8.5 or above. Before surgery, it is typical that HIV-positive

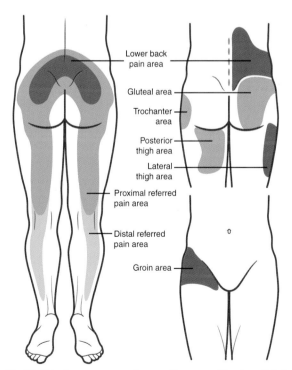

Fig. 5.4 Pain diagram representing possible areas of facet-mediated referred pain.

people should have a negative viral titer. Although hepatitis C is no longer a contraindication for a posterior fusion due to the availability of oral antiviral medications, it is typical for patients to be tested for the virus before surgery. Before considering surgery, patients with a BMI of 50 or more will be directed to a nutritionist and, potentially, a bariatric surgeon.

Preoperative Workup

Patients under the age of 40 who are relatively healthy and have no medical problems usually only require a cursory examination. Surgical blood work is frequently requested before surgery. A pregnancy test and urinalysis will be required of female patients. Physicians may request medical clearance from a trained perioperative physician for persons over the age of 40, in addition to blood work. Patients are given preoperative documentation that states that they should not eat or drink anything after midnight the night before the surgery. Patients must also stop taking any antiinflammatory or blood thinner medications for 10 days before surgery (with the approval of the prescribing physician). There are also a variety of herbal supplements that can raise the risk of bleeding, and patients are asked to stop taking these. Patients are also asked to stop smoking 2 weeks before surgery and for up to 2 years afterward.

The patient is seen in the office for a final consultation after being preoperatively examined and worked up. Before surgery, the physician should examine the patient, obtain medical clearance, and address any remaining questions. If mobility listhesis is suspected, lumbar flexion and extension x-rays are frequently sought before surgery.

Procedural Technique

There are several different methods for accomplishing posterior fusion; however, this section will focus on the FacetCore Fusion System[12] used in combination with the 3D GraftRasp System[13] from SurGenTec, LLC. It is critical to execute appropriate decortication of the bone and employ an adequate volume of bone graft once the facet allograft is implanted, for fusion to occur. If required, the rasp can be used to decorticate directly over the facet joints and transverse processes.

For bone to develop and optimal fusion to occur, a bone graft must be placed directly over the decorticated area.

The patient is positioned in prone on a radiolucent table (Fig. 5.5) with the lumbar spine slightly flexed so that the spine is in a neutral position and the facet joints may be seen on imaging. To properly position the patient and achieve optimal fluoroscopic imaging, a radiolucent pain table with gel rolls (optional) is recommended.

Surgical Steps

CORTICAL ALLOGRAFT IMPLANT PLACEMENT WITH FACETCORE FUSION SYSTEM

1. An approximately 1-inch incision is made bilaterally, one fingerbreadth lateral to the facets or directly over the facet joint (Fig. 5.6).
2. The facet joint is located with a guidewire and imaging (Fig. 5.7).
3. A facet locator is then inserted over the guidewire into the facet joint (Fig. 5.8).
4. A drill guide is docked on the facet joint (Fig. 5.9).
5. An orthopedic drill is used to prepare the insertion site (Fig. 5.10).
6. The cortical allograft implant is inserted into facet joint (Fig. 5.11).
7. The GraftRasp is used to decorticate the facet joint and deliver bone graft to the bleeding bone[9] (Fig. 5.12).
8. Steps 2 to 7 are then repeated on the contralateral side.

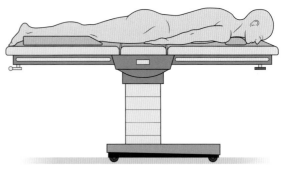

Fig. 5.5 Prone position. Anesthesia: local with sedation or general anesthesia. Anticipated timing: 30 to 60 minutes.

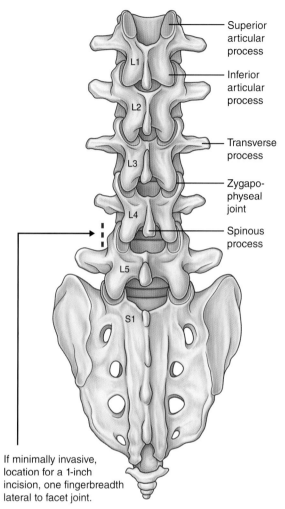

Superior articular process

Inferior articular process

Transverse process

Zygapo-physeal joint

Spinous process

If minimally invasive, location for a 1-inch incision, one fingerbreadth lateral to facet joint.

Fig. 5.6 Incision and lumbar anatomy.[12]

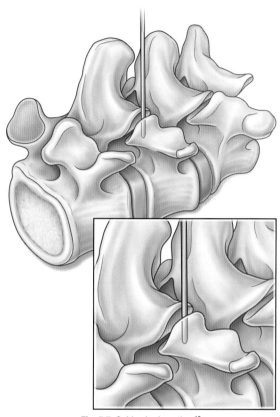

Fig. 5.7 Guidewire insertion.[12]

Postoperative Management

Postoperative: One week after surgery, patients are seen again. They must wear a lumbar sacral orthosis (LSO) brace after surgery for at least 6 weeks, but no more than 8 weeks, as this can cause back deconditioning. For the first 6 weeks, no lifting of more than 5 pounds is permitted. Showering is permitted 72 hours following surgery, with water running over the incision if it is covered by Steri-Strips. Patients are tested for allergies and given antibiotics

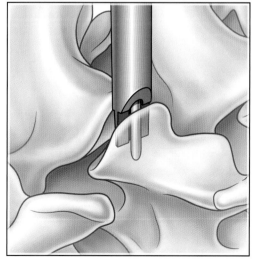

Fig. 5.8 Facet locator placed into the facet joint.[12]

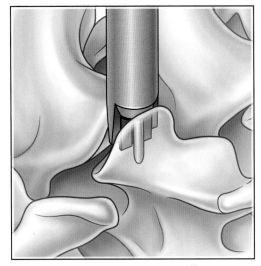

Fig. 5.9 Drill guide placement.[12]

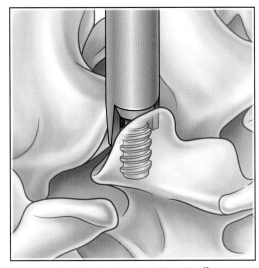

Fig. 5.11 Cortical allograft insertion.[12]

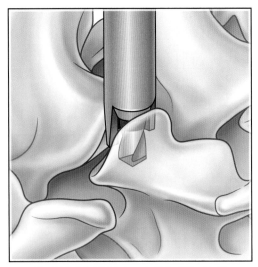

Fig. 5.10 Drill bit fully inserted into drill guide.[12]

after surgery. Cephalexin (Keflex) 500 mg four times a day for 3 days is commonly recommended. Patients will also receive postoperative narcotic medication.[14]

Six weeks: At the 6-week visit the brace is discontinued. The patient can now lift up to 15 pounds but nothing more.

Three months: At the 3-month postoperative follow-up, anteroposterior (AP)/lateral x-rays

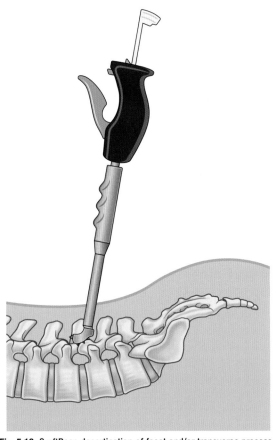

Fig. 5.12 GraftRasp decortication of facet and/or transverse process.

may be taken at the physician's discretion. At this visit we may begin to see bony callus formation. A bone growth stimulator is often requested at this time to help augment the fusion.

Six months: At the 6-month postoperative follow-up, the patient receives a repeat set of x-rays of the lumbar spine.

One year: The patient is seen 1-year postoperative. If the patient is doing well with no complaints, they may be discharged. If pain is lingering, x-rays are taken along with a CT scan to assess fusion.

Potential Complications

Every visit should include taking the patient's temperature and assessing and evaluating the incision. If the patient has a fever or the incision appears reddish or irritated, a more thorough examination is required to rule out the risk of infection. Soft tissue infections or septic arthritis are uncommon with this procedure, given its minimal access and sterile technique.[15] Additionally, the anesthesia department will administer prophylactic preoperative antibiotics to the patient before the incision. Depending on the patient's weight and allergies, the doctor may prescribe 1 to 2 g of cefazolin (Ancef).

- **Facet fracture**: Facet fractures are a possibility. This is a rare and infrequent occurrence. If a unilateral facet fracture occurs, the allograft implant and bone graft should be used to keep the facet stable. It is also necessary to achieve intertransverse fusion between the transverse processes. A brace will be worn by the patient, and a bone development stimulant should be administered.
- **Cerebrospinal fluid leak**: A cerebrospinal fluid (CSF) leak is a rare occurrence but can happen if the guidewire is inserted into the dural canal. Patients with postsurgical headaches should be evaluated for a possible CSF leak—if the patient develops a postural headache following the procedure, this is usually a red flag. Observation, a blood patch, or a formal surgical closure are all options for treatment.
- **Hematoma**: A hematoma will be benign if it occurs in the subfascial layer without any physical decompression of the neural components. Over

time, the hematoma will normally dissolve on its own.
- **Damage to the nerve root**: This is a highly unlikely situation. This is best avoided by staying within the facet joint and out of the neural foramen during surgery.
- **Nonunion**: In both instrumented and noninstrumented fusions, nonunion can occur. The failure of a posterolateral intertransverse and facet fusion to heal does not exclude the patient from undergoing additional surgeries, and the patient can expect to have an exploration of fusion and revision without disrupting the previous operation. This technique allows physicians to generate several surface areas between bleeding bone and bone graft, providing patients with the highest chance of successful fusion through improved bone preparation and graft placement. Minimal soft tissue disturbance and a lower likelihood of neurologic deficiency are two major benefits of this method.

Conclusion

Facet fusion is a technique that has been used for more than half a century. Modern medical technology has improved results. New treatments and techniques allow for lumbar spine stabilization and fusion without the use of hardware and with a less intrusive approach.

REFERENCES

1. Virk S, Qureshi S, Sandhu H. History of spinal fusion: where we came from and where we are going. *HSS J.* 2020;16(2):137-142.
2. Rajasekaran S, Naresh-Babu J. Translaminar facetal screw (Magerl's) fixation. *Neurol India.* 2005;53(4):520-524.
3. Peek RD, Wiltse LL. History of spinal fusion. In: Cotler JM, Cotler HB, eds. *Spinal Fusion.* New York, NY: Springer; 2010. Available at: https://doi.org/10.1007/978-1-4612-3272-8_1.
4. Verdecia FD, Medina HM. Percutaneous fusion of lumbar facet with bone allograft. *Coluna/Columna.* 2015;14:37-40. https://www.scielo.br/j/coluna/a/fBzmCR3r3jdhnLfVHLwM6ph/?lang=en&format=pdf
5. Canto FR, Garcia SB, Issa JP, et al. Influence of decortication of the recipient graft bed on graft integration and tissue neoformation in the graft-recipient bed interface. *Eur Spine J.* 2008;17(5):706-714.
6. Manchikanti L, Pampati V, Rivera J, Fellows B, Beyer C, Damron K. Role of facet joints in chronic low back pain in the elderly: a controlled comparative prevalence study. 2001;1(4):332-337. onlinelibrary.wiley.com/doi/epdf/10.1046/j.1533-2500.2001.01034.x.

7. Perolat R, Kastler A, Nicot B, et al. Facet joint syndrome: from diagnosis to interventional management. *Insights Imaging.* 2018;9(5):773-789.
8. Yan YZ, Li QP, Wu CC, et al. Rate of presence of 11 thoracic vertebrae and 6 lumbar vertebrae in asymptomatic Chinese adult volunteers. *J Orthop Surg Res.* 2018;13(1):124.
9. Dunlop RB, Adams MA, Hutton WC. Disc space narrowing and the lumbar facet joints. *J Bone Joint Surg Br.* 1984;66(5):706-710.
10. Inoue N, Orías AAE, Segami K. Biomechanics of the lumbar facet joint. *Spine Surg Relat Res.* 2019;4(1):1-7.
11. Mooney V, Robertson J. The facet syndrome. *Clin Orthop Relat Res.* 1976;(115):149-156.
12. FacetCoreTM Fusion System. Surgical Technique Guide. *Boca Raton: SurGenTec LLC*; 2021.
13. The 3D GraftRasp System. Surgical Technique Guide. *Boca Raton: SurGenTec LLC*; 2021.
14. Bajwa SJ, Haldar R. Pain management following spinal surgeries: an appraisal of the available options. *J Craniovertebr Junction Spine.* 2015;6(3):105-110.
15. Mueller K, Zhao D, Johnson O, et al. The difference in surgical site infection rates between open and minimally invasive spine surgery for degenerative lumbar pathology: a retrospective single center experience of 1442 cases. *Oper Neurosurg (Hagerstown).* 2019;16(6):750-755.

Chapter 6

Posterior Spinal Fusion

Ryan Budwany, Michael A. Fishman, Alaa Abd-Elsayed, and
Steven M. Falowski

The many etiologies of degenerative lumbar spinal stenosis include hypertrophied ligamentum flavum, osteophytes, facet joint hypertrophy, and degeneration of the disc space.[1] The burden of these accumulated degenerative changes often leads to lumbar spinal stenosis, which can occur earlier in those born with a congenitally narrow canal.[2] Although the major culprit is the aging spine, the cascade of these degenerative changes and stenosis is amplified by the combination of these mentioned factors.

At present there are several treatment options for those with spinal stenosis, as well as for those with degenerative changes, and these range from conservative measures to surgical treatments. Conservative measures may include physical therapy, medications, and epidural steroid injections and are generally reserved for those with mild or moderate symptoms but can also be used with those who demonstrate further progression.[3] More invasive options, such as open laminectomy or decompression of the neural structures with or without transpedicular screw fixation, have been the main option for the management of patients in whom conservative measures fail.[4] However, surgical therapy may not be optimal in some cases, such as in patients with medical comorbidities. In addition, open decompression and fusion can be associated with prolonged recovery time, and surgical complications, such as cerebrospinal fluid leak, nerve injury, deep wound infections, misplaced hardware, and hardware failures, may result.[5] It is well documented that despite best efforts with multimodal management, chronic back pain may develop, resulting in postlaminectomy syndrome.[5,6] The association of posterior lateral fusion with altered spinal dynamics is also well documented, and this can lead to adjacent segment disease and degeneration.[7] Because of these

limitations, minimally invasive options with reduced procedural risks should be considered.

Research into the use of interspinous spacers (IPS) in indirect decompression has shown positive outcomes with a favorable risk profile in the treatment of lumbar spinal stenosis. The implantation of IPS limits extension in patients with stenosis who display symptoms of neurogenic claudication that is relieved in flexion.[8] However, its use is limited in that these cases are often associated with degenerative changes, spondylolisthesis, and multiple pain generators such as disc degeneration and facet joint hypertrophy, which is not treated by indirect decompression.

Novel strategies for management of these patients with the use of minimally invasive devices for interspinous fixation (ISF) can address both the stenosis and degeneration and offer an option to patients that will result in decreased morbidity with the potential for equal or comparable efficacy to open surgical decompression with or without fusion. Mechanically, these devices stabilize the adjacent spinous processes and decompress neural structures by blocking extension, minimizing altered spinal dynamics and the risk of adjacent segment disease. Biomechanically, ISF provides immediate flexion-extension balance and effective stabilization for arthrodesis while preserving motion.[9,10] Proper patient selection leads to the inclusion of patients with moderate to severe spinal stenosis who have signs and symptoms of neurogenic claudication. Other symptoms may include back and leg pain. ISF is a viable, minimally invasive treatment option for those patients not suited for pedicle screw fixation, such as those with medical comorbidities or advanced age, as well as those considered earlier in the treatment paradigm who are either considered too young for traditional surgery or wish to avoid traditional open surgical treatment.

TABLE 6.1   **Common Indications and Contraindications**[1,2,5-9,11]

Indications	Major Contraindications
For use in the noncervical spine (T1–S1). With fixation/attachment to the spinous process in the following patient conditions: • Spondylolisthesis • Radiculopathy • Neurogenic claudication • Chronic back pain • Degenerative disc disease • Spondylosis	• Active infection • Allergy or sensitivity to titanium • Patients who are immunocompromised • Fracture or lack of spinous process • Anatomic deficit in the lamina or posterior arch (i.e., laminectomy, pars defect, or prior fusion at level[s] to be treated)

Patients undergoing ISF are treated similarly to those undergoing other surgical procedures, with perioperative workup including lab work, and cessation of anticoagulants. Postoperative care involves limitation in activity for 2 to 6 weeks, wound care, and associated follow ups.

Advantages of ISF over pedicle screw fixation include, but are not limited to, minimal invasiveness of skin and muscle, reduced operative times, and favorable efficacy with reference to visual analog scale (VAS) and Oswestry Disability Index (ODI) scores at 1-year follow-up.[11] There are several devices on the market; these may vary in terms of application and patient selection and may coincide with or without a decompression or anterior spinal fusion. A typical stand-alone ISF device (for the treatment of lumbar spinal stenosis and degenerative disease) is demonstrated in this chapter. Common indications and contraindications are listed in Table 6.1. The procedure is performed as follows:

Step 1: Start with the patient in the supine position. The use of a lumbar roll is suggested to minimize lumbar lordosis.

Step 2: Identify landmarks at the appropriate level. Prepare the skin and inject local anesthetic into the skin.

Step 3: After retracting the skin, muscle dissection is taken down to the spinolaminar junctions on both sides, exposing the full spinous process. The rongeur is used to resect a segment of the supraspinous ligament and remove the interspinous ligament (Fig. 6.1).

Step 4: Spread the sizer to the approximate diameter of the barrel (Fig. 6.2).

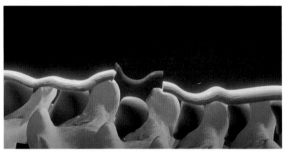

Fig. 6.1 Removal of interspinous ligament, maintaining the bony structure of the spinous process.

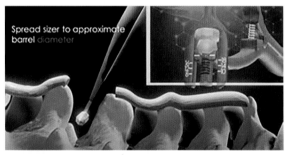

Spread sizer to approximate barrel diameter

Fig. 6.2 Use of sizer to determine barrel size of implant and use as a reamer to prepare the bony surface for fusion.

Step 5: Use the ratcheting feature to measure the space and lock at the desired measurement (Fig. 6.3).

Step 6: Note the plate size; the scale on the diagram in Fig. 6.3 indicates the plate size.

Compare the plate size with the locator to determine the plate length (Fig. 6.4A–C).

Step 7: The implant is prepared in the grafting station.

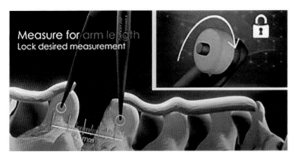

Fig. 6.3 Determining the length of the implant.

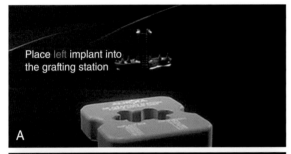

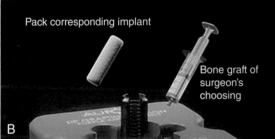

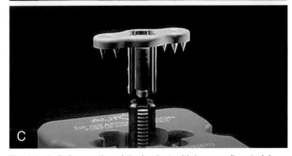

Fig. 6.4 (A–C) Preparation of the implant with bone graft material.

Step 8: Place implant in the interspinous space to the spinolaminar junction and compress onto the spinous processes (Fig. 6.5A,B).

Step 9: Place the bone graft material around the graft and bony surfaces (Fig. 6.6).

Step 10: Muscle and skin incision closure with sutures (Fig. 6.7A,B).

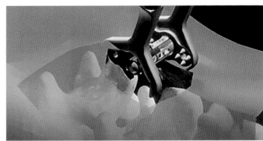

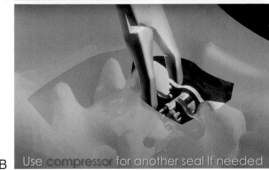

Fig. 6.5 (A, B) Placement of implant.

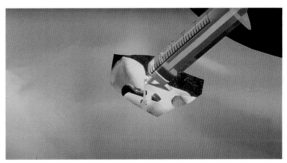

Fig. 6.6 Injecting bone graft material.

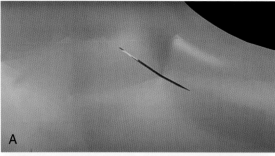

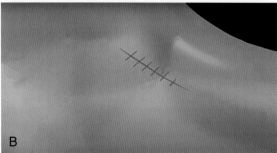

Fig. 6.7 (A) Incision site. (B) Skin closure.

REFERENCES

1. Zaina F, Tomkins-Lane C, Carragee E, et al. Surgical versus non-surgical treatment for lumbar spinal stenosis. *Cochrane Database Syst Rev.* 2016;1:CD010264.
2. Siebert E, Pruss H, Klingebiel R, Failli V, Einhaupl KM, Schwab JM. Lumbar spinal stenosis: syndrome, diagnostics and treatment. *Nat Rev Neurol.* 2009;5(7):392-403.
3. Backstrom KM, Whitman JM, Flynn TW. Lumbar spinal stenosis-diagnosis and management of the aging spine. *Man Ther.* 2011;16(4):308-317.
4. Bridwell KH, Sedgewick TA, O'Brien MF, Lenke LG, Baldus C. The role of fusion and instrumentation in the treatment of degenerative spondylolisthesis with spinal stenosis. *J Spinal Disord.* 1993;6:461-472.
5. Esses SI, Sachs BL, Dreyzin V. Complications associated with the technique of pedicle screw fixation. A selected survey of ABS members. *Spine.* 1993;18:2231-2238; discussion 2239.
6. Jutte PC, Castelein RM. Complications of pedicle screws in lumbar and lumbosacral fusions in 105 consecutive primary operations. *Eur Spine J.* 2002;11:594-598.
7. Hilibrand AS, Robbins M. Adjacent segment degeneration and adjacent segment disease: the consequences of spinal fusion? *Spine J.* 2004;4:190S-194S.
8. Nunley PD, Patel VV, Orndorff DG, Lavelle WF, Block JE, Geisler FH. Five-year durability of stand-alone interspinous process decompression for lumbar spinal stenosis. *Clin Interv Aging.* 2017;12:1409-1417.
9. Gonzalez-Blohm SA, Doulgeris JJ, Kamran Aghayev WE, et al. Biomechanical analysis of an interspinous fusion device as a stand-alone and as supplemental fixation to posterior expandable interbody cages in the lumbar spine. *J Neurosurg Spine.* 2014;20(2):209-219.
10. Karahalios DG, Musacchio MJ. Lumbar interspinous devices: fusion and motion sparing. In: Holly L, Anderson P, eds. *Essentials of Spinal Stabilization.* Cham: Springer; 2017.
11. Kim HJ, Bak KH, Chun HJ, et al. Posterior interspinous fusion device for one-level fusion in degenerative lumbar spine disease: comparison with pedicle screw fixation - preliminary report of at least one year follow up. *J Korean Neurosurg Soc.* 2012;52(4):359-364.

Chapter 7

Interspinous Fusion With Lateral Percutaneous Technique

Michael Gyorfi, Steven M. Falowski, and Alaa Abd-Elsayed

Introduction

The lateral percutaneous technique is a minimally invasive approach to interspinous-interlaminar fusion with a device used to stabilize the thoracic, lumbar, and sacral spine. It is intended for usage with bone graft material placed into the device and is designed for connection to the posterior noncervical spine at the spinous processes in the interspinous space through its bilateral locking plates. This lateral minimally invasive surgery (MIS) technique is performed under fluoroscopy. A wide variety of sizes allows for improved anatomic fit, and the core threaded post provides regulated distraction.

Indications

The intended use of the lateral percutaneous technique is with a posterior, nonpedicle supplemental fixation device at a single level in the noncervical spine. It is designed to fixate/attach plates to spinous processes to achieve supplementary fusion within the interspinous space. The most common indications are degenerative disc disease (DDD), spondylolisthesis, and spinal trauma.[1]

Patient Selection

Proper patient selection may greatly affect the efficacy. Smoking has been shown to increase the incidence of nonunion. These patients should be encouraged to stop smoking and be made aware of the increased risk. Patients who are alcoholic, malnourished, or obese are also at an elevated risk for complications. Lastly, osteoporosis may make patients more prone to poorer outcomes and complications such as spinous process fractures.

Step by Step Description of the Procedure

1. Preoperative planning is the first step. Routine preoperative tests include anteroposterior (AP) and lateral x-rays (flexion and extension views are also indicated), magnetic resonance imaging (MRI), and/or computed tomography (CT) myelography. Gross instability, severe spondylolisthesis, major scoliosis, severe osteoporosis, and ankylosed spinal section must all be ruled out. A preoperative CT is advised if the lateral MIS approach is necessary at L3–L4 or above, to ensure a safe trajectory.
2. The patient should be positioned in a prone posture on a frame that reduces lordosis and prevents the abdomen from being squeezed. Tilting the pelvis by inclining the table at the level of the pelvis is recommended. The result will be that the spinous processes are naturally distracted. In both the AP and lateral planes, the frame and operating table must be radiolucent. The lateral decubitus position may be used as an alternative patient position (Fig. 7.1).
3. Identify the midline of the spinous processes at the level to be instrumented using manual palpation and AP fluoroscopy and insert a spinal needle. Define anatomic landmarks and transfer them onto the skin using lateral fluoroscopy. The superior margin of the inferior spinous process is marked by a skin mark (Fig. 7.2; seen in blue). The inferior border of the superior spinous process is marked by a second skin mark (shown in magenta). The posterior boundary

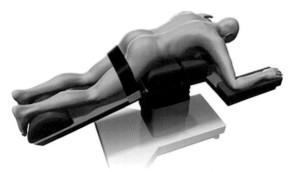

Fig. 7.1 Prone patient positioning.

of the facet joint is marked with a third skin mark (shown in orange). Make a 2.5-cm longitudinal incision between the blue and magenta lines and along the orange line (Fig. 7.2).

4. Insert the guidewire into the aiming device until the first stop is reached. The guidewire is introduced through the incision. The guidewire should be put as far anterior as feasible for best results. Increase the guidewire length by depressing the aiming device knob. Carefully move the guidewire between the spinous processes and puncture the interspinous ligament under lateral fluoroscopy (Fig. 7.3).

5. Advance the guidewire about 2 cm across the midline of the spine under AP fluoroscopy. With AP and lateral views, double-check the location of the guidewire (Fig. 7.4).

6. Remove the aiming device from the guidewire by depressing the aiming device knob. It is critical to keep the guidewire in place. Thread the guidewire extension onto the guidewire. While inserting dilators, sleeves, and other devices, the guidewire extension assists in maintaining proper guidewire placement (Fig. 7.5).

7. Over the guidewire, slide the 3-mm soft tissue dilator. The 3-mm dilator is introduced through the skin incision while holding the guidewire in place under AP fluoroscopy. Rotate and advance the 3-mm dilator until it is near to the spinous processes. Optional: If facet hypertrophy prevents the sleeve from docking against the spinous processes, the bone rasp can be placed over the guidewire and turned clockwise to progressively diminish the facets' bulk. Leave the guidewire in place while removing the bone rasp. Optional: If the soft tissue rasp is unable to proceed between the spinous processes because it is in contact with them, the starter rasp can be put over the guidewire and spun clockwise to gradually divert the spinous processes (Fig. 7.6).

8. The soft tissue rasp is introduced into the interspinous process space over the guidewire. The interspinous ligament is partially removed, and the spinous processes are partially decorticated by rotating the rasp clockwise. After that, the rasp is removed, but the guidewire is left in place (Fig. 7.7).

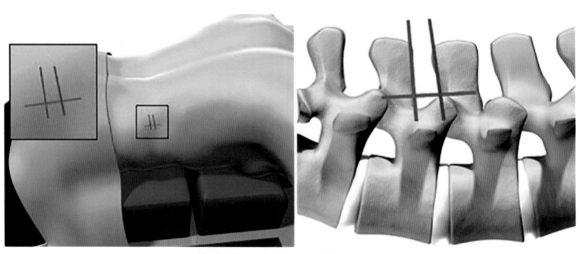

Fig. 7.2 Demonstrating anatomic landmarks.

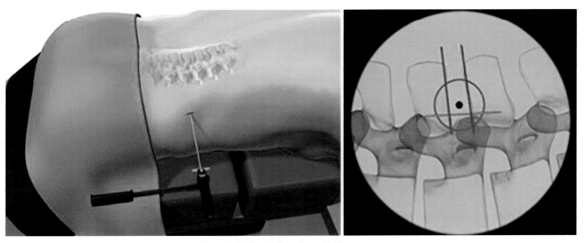

Fig. 7.3 Guidewire insertion with fluoroscopy.

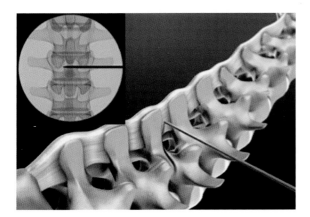

Fig. 7.4 Advancement of guidewire.

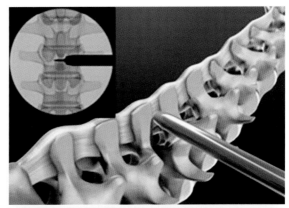

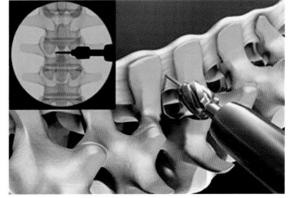

Fig. 7.6 Start of rasp insertion.

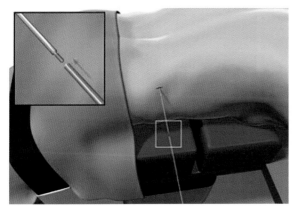

Fig. 7.5 Aiming device removal.

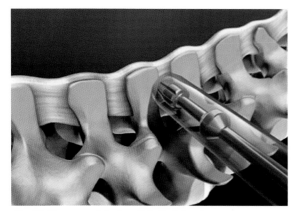

Fig. 7.7 Tissue rasp introduced into the interspinous process space.

9. Over the extended guidewire, the graduated tap is inserted. The tap is inserted clockwise into the interspinous process space under AP fluoroscopy. Engage the threads of the tap with the spinous processes with moderate effort. The spinous processes are increasingly distracted as the tap is progressed. The degree of distraction may be evaluated by looking at which tap size hole is positioned between the spinous processes once enough distraction has been achieved. The optimum implant size is determined by the degree of distraction. Leave the graduated tap in place when putting the implant onto the G2-inserter to preserve the appropriate route for implant placement (Fig. 7.8).

10. The tap includes sizing holes that correlate to the degree of distraction, and these holes may

be seen on AP fluoroscopy to estimate the implant size. The 23-mm sleeve should be slid over the 20-mm sleeve. The 23-mm sleeve should be inserted until it is close to the spinous processes. For the 26-mm sleeve, repeat the process. Remove the 20-mm and 23-mm sleeves but keep the 26-mm sleeve (Fig. 7.9).

11. Remove the guidewire while leaving the sleeve in place against the lateral surface of the spinous processes. Attach the relevant size insertion adapter to the distal end of the inserter after determining the appropriate size. The insertion adapter will be the same color as the hex nut of the same size (Fig. 7.10).

12. To attach the device, make sure the inserter is unlocked. The position indicator should be aligned with the arrowhead (Fig. 7.11).

13. The spring-loaded adapter shaft is first squeezed against the fixed plate knob until it bottoms out, then turned counterclockwise for about one-eighth of a full turn (Fig. 7.12).

14. Snap the implant into place by aligning the extension plate in the same orientation as the laser engraving. The extension plate can be aligned with the plate reference lines with proper positioning (Fig. 7.13).

15. Rotate the plunger knob clockwise until the position indicator is in the locked position to secure the device to the inserter. The device is automatically locked to the inserter when the plunger stop clicks to the right (Fig. 7.14).

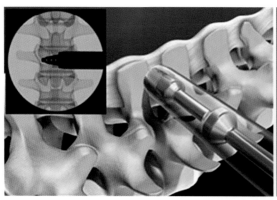
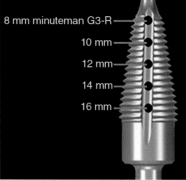

Fig. 7.8 Graduated tip insertion.

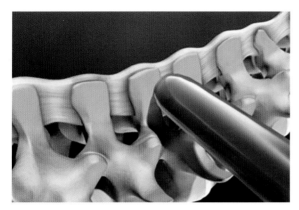

Fig. 7.9 A 23-mm sleeve sliding over the 20-mm sleeve.

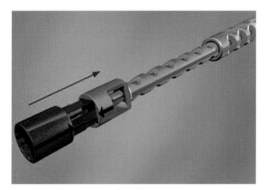

Fig. 7.10 Insertion adaptor attachment.

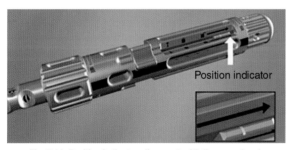

Fig. 7.11 Position indicator alignment with the arrowhead.

Position indicator

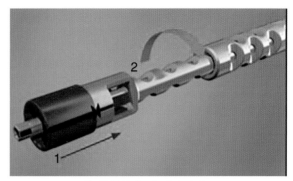

Fig. 7.12 Spring-loaded adaptor.

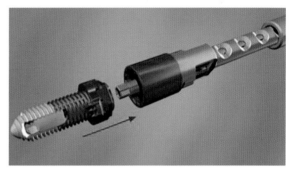

Fig. 7.13 Attaching the extension plate.

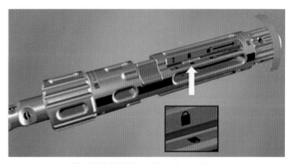

Fig. 7.14 Rotation of the plunger knob.

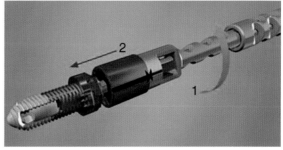

Fig. 7.15 The hex nut engagement with the insertion adaptor.

16. Hold the fixed plate knob and (1) spin the adaptor shaft clockwise about one-eighth of a turn, and (2) gently spring forward the adaptor shaft. The hex nut will be engaged by the insertion adaptor. Slowly twist the adaptor shaft until the insertion adaptor slips into position if it does not correctly contact the hex nut (Fig. 7.15).

17. Bone graft material is introduced by threading bone graft material into the threaded body while holding one wing open and the other closed. The devices external threads are likewise covered with bone graft material (Fig. 7.16).

18. The inserter is inserted into the sleeve with the device connected and progresses to the interspinous process area, aiming as far anterior as feasible. To engage the threads, rotate the inserter clockwise. The device is moved into the interspinous space under fluoroscopy until the fixed plate reaches the spinous processes (Fig. 7.17).

19. To use the extension plate, first slide and hold the plunger stop to the left, then turn the plunger knob clockwise until it stops. The plate deployment symbol will be near to the position indicator (Fig. 7.18).

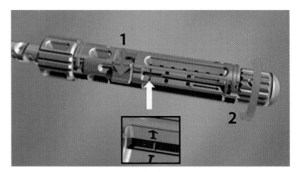

Fig. 7.18 Extension plate.

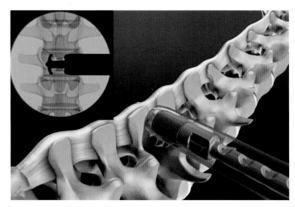

Fig. 7.19 Extension plate deployment.

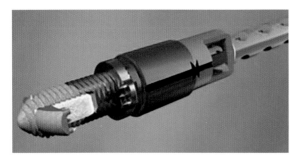

Fig. 7.16 Bone graft material inserted into the threaded body.

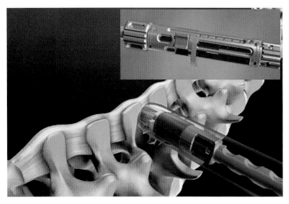

Fig. 7.17 G2 insertion into the sleeve.

20. Ensure that the extension plate has been deployed and will contact the spinous processes as far anterior as feasible during fixation using fluoroscopy. The device may now be attached to the spinous processes (Fig. 7.19).

21. To secure the implant to the spinous processes, hold the inserter in place and advance the fixed plate by rotating the fixed plate knob clockwise. The extension plate will be brought to contact the distal lateral surface of the spinous processes as the fixed plate is tightened (Fig. 7.20).

22. A ratcheting sensation will be felt, which represents the implant's locking mechanism. The amount of torque used should be proportional to the patient's bone quality. Check the plate reference lines on the inserter to ensure appropriate extension plate alignment during fixation (Fig. 7.21).

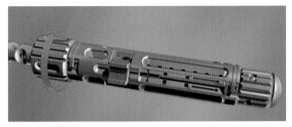

Fig. 7.20 Fixed plate advancement.

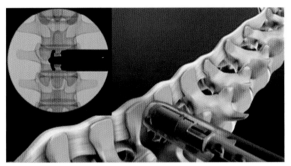

Fig. 7.21 Implant locking mechanism.

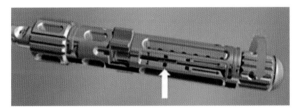

Fig. 7.22 Rotation of the plunger knob.

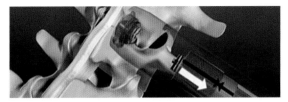

Fig. 7.23 Implant body removal.

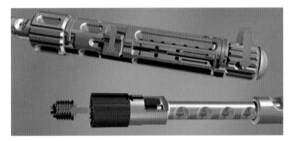

Fig. 7.24 Removal of inserter body.

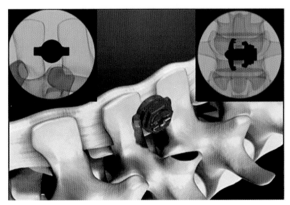

Fig. 7.25 Completed interspinous fusion.

23. Twist the plunger knob counterclockwise until the position indicator reaches the locked position. The plunger stop moves to the right automatically (Fig. 7.22).
24. To detach the removable body from the implant, gently pull the inserter laterally. The inserter is taken out of the patient's body (Fig. 7.23).
25. Slide and hold the plunger stop back to the left once outside the patient's body, then spin the plunger knob counterclockwise until it stops. The inserter's removable body is now detachable (Fig. 7.24).
26. The sleeve is taken off. Sutures or Steri-Strips are then used to close the wound (Fig. 7.25).

Contraindications

The lateral percutaneous technique for interspinous fusion is designed for the majority of patients; however, there are contraindications such as spinal anatomy or disease that would cause the device to be unstable and/or prevent implantation, the most common being severe osteoporosis, scoliosis, infection, and acute fracture of the pars interarticularis or spinous process. Other contraindications are pregnancy and an allergy to titanium alloy.

Complications

The most common adverse effects or complications related to this technique include the implant being malpositioned, failure of the procedure to improve symptoms, implant migration, spinous process fractures, and mechanical failure of the device. Surgical-related complications include, but are not limited to, myocardial infarction, infection, deep vein thrombosis, hematoma, spinal cord injury, pneumonia, wound dehiscence, and/or pain at the operative site.

REFERENCES

1. Chan AK, Bisson EF, Bydon M, et al. A comparison of minimally invasive transforaminal lumbar interbody fusion and decompression alone for degenerative lumbar spondylolisthesis. *Neurosurg Focus.* 2019;46(5):E13.

Chapter 8

Measuring Outcomes

Ryan Steven D'Souza, Mayank Gupta, and Alaa Abd-Elsayed

Introduction

The assessment of pain is complex and challenging. It is crucial that clinicians and researchers use validated instruments in the assessment of pain-related outcomes. Given the multifaceted and complex nature of pain, there is no one single measure that captures the pain experience. Instead, scales that measure pain intensity, pain quality, psychosocial impact, emotional functioning, and physical functioning can be used. In this chapter, we review the most commonly used pain assessment tools in both the clinical and the research setting.

Pain Intensity

SELF-REPORT SCALES

Pain intensity is one of the most common aspects of pain that clinicians and researchers ask patients to rate when measuring pain-related outcomes. Although reliability and reproducibility may vary at different times in the same patient, the ease, speed, and importance of a measure of pain intensity when assessing outcomes highlights its relevance. Self-report scales are the most frequently used type of pain intensity scale. These include the numeric rating scale (NRS), visual analog scale (VAS), verbal rating scale (VRS), and other self-report scales (e.g., pain drawing measures).

The NRS can be presented in an oral or written format, and patients are asked to rate their pain on a scale of 0 to 10, with 0 signifying no pain at all and 10 signifying the worst pain imaginable.[1] Sometimes, ranges of 0 to 20 or 0 to 100 are utilized. Although there is no consensus on clinically significant changes, some consider a 2-point decrease on the NRS to be a clinically significant change in pain intensity.[2] The major advantages of the NRS are that it is quick and easy to administer and has a very high completion rate among respondents.[1]

Similar to the NRS, the VAS employs a quantitative method of rating pain intensity. It utilizes a 10-cm line with end points signifying no pain at all at one end (0 cm) and the worst pain imaginable at the other end (10 cm). Patients place a mark at a point along the line that characterizes their pain intensity. Lower completion rates are seen with VAS scales compared with NRS scales.[3,4]

The VRS includes a list of descriptive words to grade pain intensity. Lists may have from 4 to 15 descriptors, and these descriptors may be assigned a value. The following is an example: 0 = no pain, 1 = mild pain, 2 = moderate pain, 3 = severe pain. Similar to the NRS, this scale is quick and easy to administer and complete, although it may be harder to administer to patients with limited vocabulary or literacy comprehension.[5]

Pain intensity scales using images may also be presented to patients. With these, the patient is asked to indicate the level of pain they are experiencing based on pictures of different facial expressions. These were developed for use with children, as well as with patients with low literacy levels. One example is the FACES scale that presents six different drawings of faces that represent six levels of pain intensity. The "very happy" face represents a score of 0, whereas the "very upset and crying" face represents a score of 10. Concerns regarding the use of this scale include that ratings may be affected by emotional reactions, and interpretation of the scales may vary between people and is affected by age, literacy, and culture.[6,7]

BEHAVIORAL SCALE

There are many types of patient to whom self-report pain intensity scales cannot be administered. These include pediatric patients who are not capable of using self-report measures, critically ill patients who are unable to communicate (e.g., intubated), and other patient populations. The inability to self-report pain does not exclude the possibility of its presence. In these settings, clinicians and researchers should utilize validated behavioral measures to assess behavioral indicators of pain intensity.

One example of a behavioral scale is the Face, Legs, Activity, Cry, and Consolability (FLACC) scale that assesses postoperative pain in children.[8] On this scale the five behaviors that are present in the title of the scale are rated, with each component rated on a 0 to 2 scale, with the maximum total questionnaire score being 10.[8]

Pain Quality

Although grading pain intensity is helpful in assessing the severity and extent of pain, other scales that provide a more in-depth measure of the quality and affective components of the pain experience are often useful. These can further help the clinician or researcher assess how the pain experience is impacting the patient.

MCGILL PAIN QUESTIONNAIRE

The McGill Pain Questionnaire (MPQ) is a tool that assesses the quality and affective component of pain. Patients choose descriptors of the pain experience from 78 potential descriptors.[9] These descriptors evaluate four separate domains: sensory, affective, evaluative, and miscellaneous. Patients also indicate the location of their pain on an anatomical drawing and provide details on alleviating and exacerbating factors. This questionnaire generates three scores: the Pain Rating Index, number of descriptor words chosen, and the pain intensity rating. This scale is widely used in the pain setting, and there is also a short version (15-item tool), the Short-Form (SF) MPQ.[10] The tool has been validated through multiple studies, and its subscales are associated with patient quality of life, analgesic medication use, and sensitivity to pain treatment.

Psychosocial Impact

Another facet of the pain experience is the behavioral and social aspect of chronic pain. Several validated instruments have been developed to quantify the pain experience across various social arenas, as well as in behavioral and interpersonal relationships.

WEST HAVEN-YALE MULTIDIMENSIONAL PAIN INVENTORY

The West Haven-Yale Multidimensional Pain Inventory (WHYMPI) is a 52-item questionnaire that employs a 7-point Likert scale and is used to assess the psychosocial and behavioral aspects of the pain experience.[11] The questionnaire is divided into three sections, with each section including several scales. The first section consists of six scales that measure pain interference in work and leisure activities, interpersonal relations, spousal support, pain severity and suffering, control over life, and negative mood. The second section measures the patient's perception of the responses to their pain elicited from their significant other. These include solicitous responses, distraction, or negative responses. The third and final section assesses the frequency with which the patient performs daily activities such as household chores, outdoor work, and social events. There are three reliable profiles that can be characterized in patients with persistent pain after completion of this questionnaire: dysfunctional, interpersonally distressed, and adaptive copers.

MINNESOTA MULTIPHASIC PERSONALITY INVENTORY

The Minnesota Multiphasic Personality Inventory (MMPI) is an objective tool to measure personality and psychological functioning.[12] The most recent iteration of this scale, known as the Minnesota Multiphasic Personality Investory-2 Restructured Form (MMPI-2-RF), includes 338 items that yield scores on 3 higher-order scales, 9 clinical scales, 8 validity scales, 14 somatic and cognitive scales, 11 externalizing/interpersonal/interest scales, and 5 personality scales.

PATIENT REPORTED OUTCOMES MEASUREMENT INFORMATION SYSTEM

The Patient Reported Outcomes Measurement Information System (PROMIS) is an initiative by the National Institutes of Health (NIH) to assess patient-reported outcomes in those with chronic diseases.[13-15] These measures cover a wide range of domains, including physical, mental, and social health, across many different medical illnesses. Pain-specific measures that are also available in this initiative include a pain interference short form, and pain intensity and behavior measures. The pain interference form contains 41 items, with four short forms ranging from 4 to 8 items each. The pain behaviors form consists of 39 items and includes a short form that has 7 items. Studies have suggested that the PROMIS pain-related scales provide comprehensive and psychometrically sound measures of pain-related outcomes, although given the novelty and recent development of PROMIS, a limited amount of evidence of their validity is currently available.

Mood and Emotional Functioning

Chronic pain is a constant stressful state and commonly coexists with mood disorders. Research has highlighted that there is considerable overlap between chronic pain and depression-induced neuroplasticity changes and both share a similar neurobiological mechanism.[16] Importantly, research has also highlighted that patients who deal with chronic pain–induced depression have a poorer prognosis than patients with chronic pain only.[16] Furthermore, chronic pain and depression together can mutually promote the severity and progression of both.

BECK DEPRESSION INVENTORY

The Beck Depression Inventory (BDI) measures emotional functioning.[17,18] This questionnaire consists of 21 items that measure the behavioral presentation of depression and assess depressive symptom severity over time. There have been two major revisions of the BDI, including the BDI-Ia and the BDI-II. The BDI-II has recently been used extensively in patients to evaluate for depression symptoms in settings with a high prevalence of pain.[17,18]

PATIENT-HEALTH QUESTIONNAIRE-9 FORM

The Patient-Health Questionnaire-9 (PHQ-9) form consists of nine items that assess for the presence and severity of depression.[19,20] Each item on the form is scored from 0 to 3, giving a total score ranging from 0 to 27. A cumulative score ≥ 10 indicates the presence of major depressive symptoms.

GENERALIZED ANXIETY DISORDER-7 FORM

The Generalized Anxiety Disorder-7 (GAD-7) form consists of seven items that assess for presence and severity

of generalized anxiety.[21,22] Each item on the form is scored from 0 to 3 giving a total score ranging from 0 to 27. Cumulative scores of 5, 10, and 15 signify mild, moderate, and severe anxiety symptoms, respectively.

PAIN ANXIETY SYMPTOMS SCALE

The Pain Anxiety Symptoms Scale (PASS) measures cognitive, physiologic, and behavioral components of pain related to fear.[23] This questionnaire consists of 53 items that are categorized into the domains of fear of pain, cognitive anxiety, somatic anxiety, avoidance, and escape. Although studies have noted the high positive predictive value of the PASS for pain-related fear, it has been criticized for having poor predictive value for disability related to pain-related fear.[24]

SHORT-FORM HEALTH SURVEY-36

The Medical Outcomes Study Short-Form Health Survey-36 (SF-36) measures a patient's perceived health status.[25,26] The SF-36 consists of 36 items that form eight separate scales including vitality, physical function, bodily pain, general health perceptions, physical role functioning, emotional role functioning, social role functioning, and mental health. The eight subscales are further combined and summarized into two domains: a physical component summary and a mental component summary. Cumulative scores range from 0 to 100, with lower scores indicating poorer health and quality of life.

Physical Conditioning and Functional Outcomes

Although some patients may continue to experience similar pain intensity and pain quality despite procedural intervention, many will note an improvement in physical conditioning and functional outcome. It is not uncommon for patients to note that their pain intensity is the same, but that they now notice that they are able to walk for longer distances, perform more household chores or yard work, and engage more in social events. Thus it is crucial to also evaluate this component of the pain experience.

OSWESTRY DISABILITY INDEX

The Oswestry Disability Index (ODI) is a common questionnaire used to evaluate functional outcomes and physical functioning in patients with acute or chronic low back pain.[27] This questionnaire yields a subjective percentage score that grades the level of physical function or disability. The cumulative score indicates the patient as functioning at a point on a range from minimal disability to bedbound. The ODI questionnaire is more effective for patients with persistent severe disability, versus the Roland-Morris Questionnaire (discussed in the following section), which is indicated more for mild to moderate disability.[28]

ROLAND-MORRIS DISABILITY QUESTIONNAIRE

The Roland-Morris Disability Questionnaire (RMQ) consists of 24 items that measure the degree of disability in patients with low back pain.[29,30] These items focus on physical activity, sleep, psychosocial features, household management, eating, and frequency of pain. The cumulative score can range from 0, indicating no disability, to 24, indicating severe disability.

Satisfaction

In certain circumstances, interventions may provide transient but not long standing relief. These may help with pain intensity, quality of life, emotional functioning, and physical functioning in the short-term, but the effects may not persist as disease and degeneration progresses. Many patients will claim that despite the effects of interventions wearing off and relief being transient, they are globally satisfied about receiving the intervention.

PATIENT GLOBAL IMPRESSION OF CHANGE

The Patient Global Impression of Change (PGIC) questionnaire reflects patient satisfaction and patient impressions regarding the efficacy of treatment or intervention.[31,32] The questionnaire is graded by a 7-point scale on which patients rate their change as very much improved, much improved, minimally improved, no change, minimally worse, much worse, or very much worse.

BRIEF PAIN INVENTORY

The Brief Pain Inventory (BPI) consists of 15 items and measures pain intensity and interference.[33] Although this questionnaire was initially developed for the cancer pain population, it is now widely used for a variety of chronic pain presentations.[34] Specifically, the questionnaire comprises pain drawings and diagrams, items regarding medications and analgesics, pain interference and intensity, relationships, mood, quality of life, and physical activities (sleep, general activity, and walking). Higher scores indicate greater severity and pain interference.[33]

Conclusion

This chapter outlines multiple validated questionnaires that span several domains to comprehensively and accurately capture the pain experience. Although certain domains may have greater relevance depending on the patient and provider, assessing pain outcomes through all domains is important, as outcomes are interrelated and impact one another.

REFERENCES

1. Younger J, McCue R, Mackey S. Pain outcomes: a brief review of instruments and techniques. *Curr Pain Headache Rep.* 2009;13(1):39-43.
2. Farrar JT, Berlin JA, Strom BL. Clinically important changes in acute pain outcome measures: a validation study. *J Pain Symptom Manage.* 2003;25(5):406-411.
3. Klimek L, Bergmann KC, Biedermann T, et al. Visual analogue scales (VAS): measuring instruments for the documentation of symptoms and therapy monitoring in cases of allergic rhinitis in everyday health care: position paper of the German Society of Allergology (AeDA) and the German Society of Allergy and Clinical Immunology (DGAKI), ENT Section, in collaboration with the working group on Clinical Immunology, Allergology and Environmental Medicine of the German Society of Otorhinolaryngology, Head and Neck Surgery (DGHNOKHC). *Allergo J Int.* 2017;26(1):16-24.
4. Delgado DA, Lambert BS, Boutris N, et al. Validation of digital visual analog scale pain scoring with a traditional paper-based visual analog scale in adults. *J Am Acad Orthop Surg Glob Res Rev.* 2018;2(3):e088.
5. Haefeli M, Elfering A. Pain assessment. *Eur Spine J.* 2006;15(suppl 1):S17-S24.
6. Li L, Liu X, Herr K. Postoperative pain intensity assessment: a comparison of four scales in Chinese adults. *Pain Med.* 2007;8(3):223-234.
7. Pathak A, Sharma S, Jensen MP. The utility and validity of pain intensity rating scales for use in developing countries. *Pain Rep.* 2018;3(5):e672.
8. Crellin DJ, Harrison D, Santamaria N, Babl FE. Systematic review of the Face, Legs, Activity, Cry and Consolability scale for assessing pain in infants and children: is it reliable, valid, and feasible for use? *Pain.* 2015;156(11):2132-2151.
9. Melzack R. The McGill Pain Questionnaire: major properties and scoring methods. *Pain.* 1975;1(3):277-299.
10. Melzack R. The short-form McGill Pain Questionnaire. *Pain.* 1987;30(2):191-197.

11. Verra ML, Angst F, Staal JB, et al. Reliability of the Multidimensional Pain Inventory and stability of the MPI classification system in chronic back pain. *BMC Musculoskelet Disord.* 2012;13:155.

12. Ruiz MA, Dorritie MT. Clinical utility of the Minnesota Multiphasic Personality Inventory-2-Restructured Form (MMPI-2-RF) in a residential treatment program for homeless individuals. *Assessment.* 2021;28(2):353-366.

13. Crins MHP, Terwee CB, Westhovens R, et al. First validation of the full PROMIS Pain Interference and Pain Behavior item banks in patients with rheumatoid arthritis. *Arthritis Care Res (Hoboken).* 2020;72(11):1550-1559.

14. St John MJ, Mitten D, Hammert WC. Efficacy of PROMIS Pain Interference and Likert Pain Scores to assess physical function. *J Hand Surg Am.* 2017;42(9):705-710.

15. Kean J, Monahan PO, Kroenke K, et al. Comparative responsiveness of the PROMIS pain interference short forms, brief pain inventory, PEG, and SF-36 bodily pain subscale. *Med Care.* 2016;54(4):414-421.

16. Sheng J, Liu S, Wang Y, Cui R, Zhang X. The link between depression and chronic pain: neural mechanisms in the brain. *Neural Plast.* 2017;2017:9724371.

17. Wang YP, Gorenstein C. Assessment of depression in medical patients: a systematic review of the utility of the Beck Depression Inventory-II. *Clinics (Sao Paulo).* 2013;68(9):1274-1287.

18. García-Batista ZE, Guerra-Peña K, Cano-Vindel A, Herrera-Martínez SX, Medrano LA. Validity and reliability of the Beck Depression Inventory (BDI-II) in general and hospital population of Dominican Republic. *PLoS One.* 2018;13(6):e0199750.

19. Levis B, Benedetti A, Thombs BD. Accuracy of Patient Health Questionnaire-9 (PHQ-9) for screening to detect major depression: individual participant data meta-analysis. *BMJ.* 2019;365:l1476.

20. Moriarty AS, Gilbody S, McMillan D, Manea L. Screening and case finding for major depressive disorder using the Patient Health Questionnaire (PHQ-9): a meta-analysis. *Gen Hosp Psychiatry.* 2015;37(6):567-576.

21. Spitzer RL, Kroenke K, Williams JB, Löwe B. A brief measure for assessing generalized anxiety disorder: the GAD-7. *Arch Intern Med.* 2006;166(10):1092-1097.

22. Johnson SU, Ulvenes PG, Øktedalen T, Hoffart A. Psychometric properties of the General Anxiety Disorder 7-Item (GAD-7) Scale in a heterogeneous psychiatric sample. *Front Psychol.* 2019;10:1713.

23. McCracken LM, Zayfert C, Gross RT. The Pain Anxiety Symptoms Scale: development and validation of a scale to measure fear of pain. *Pain.* 1992;50(1):67-73.

24. Brede E, Mayer TG, Neblett R, Williams M, Gatchel RJ. The Pain Anxiety Symptoms Scale fails to discriminate pain or anxiety in a chronic disabling occupational musculoskeletal disorder population. *Pain Pract.* 2011;11(5):430-438.

25. Lins L, Carvalho FM. SF-36 total score as a single measure of health-related quality of life: scoping review. *SAGE Open Med.* 2016;4.

26. Jenkinson C, Coulter A, Wright L. Short form 36 (SF36) health survey questionnaire: normative data for adults of working age. *BMJ.* 1993;306(6890):1437-1440.

27. Vianin M. Psychometric properties and clinical usefulness of the Oswestry Disability Index. *J Chiropr Med.* 2008;7(4):161-163.

28. Grönblad M, Hupli M, Wennerstrand P, et al. Intercorrelation and test-retest reliability of the Pain Disability Index (PDI) and the Oswestry Disability Questionnaire (ODQ) and their correlation with pain intensity in low back pain patients. *Clin J Pain.* 1993;9(3):189-195.

29. Stevens ML, Lin CC, Maher CG. The Roland Morris Disability Questionnaire. *J Physiother.* 2016;62(2):116.

30. Yamato TP, Maher CG, Saragiotto BT, Catley MJ, McAuley JH. The Roland-Morris Disability Questionnaire: one or more dimensions? *Eur Spine J.* 2017;26(2):301-308.

31. Rampakakis E, Ste-Marie PA, Sampalis JS, Karellis A, Shir Y, Fitzcharles MA. Real-life assessment of the validity of patient global impression of change in fibromyalgia. *RMD Open.* 2015;1(1):e000146.

32. Perrot S, Lantéri-Minet M. Patients' Global Impression of Change in the management of peripheral neuropathic pain: clinical relevance and correlations in daily practice. *Eur J Pain.* 2019;23(6):1117-1128.

33. Poquet N, Lin C. The Brief Pain Inventory (BPI). *J Physiother.* 2016;62(1):52.

34. Keller S, Bann CM, Dodd SL, Schein J, Mendoza TR, Cleeland CS. Validity of the brief pain inventory for use in documenting the outcomes of patients with noncancer pain. *Clin J Pain.* 2004;20(5):309-318.

INDEX

Page numbers followed by *f* and *t* indicate figures and tables, respectively.